T0316640

THE ESSENCE OF BUDO

Books by Dave Lowry

Autumn Lightning
In the Dojo
The Karate Way
Sword and Brush

THE ESSENCE OF
BUDO

A Practitioner's Guide to Understanding
the Japanese Martial Ways

DAVE LOWRY

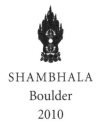

SHAMBHALA
Boulder
2010

For Meik, whose counsel and advice have always been in inverse
proportion to the quality of his jokes and puns

Shambhala Publications, Inc.
2129 13th Street
Boulder, Colorado 80302
www.shambhala.com

Printed in the United States of America

Shambhala Publications makes every effort to print on acid-free, recycled
paper.

Shambhala Publications is distributed worldwide by
Penguin Random House, Inc., and its subsidiaries.

Library of Congress Cataloging-in-Publication Data
Lowry, Dave.
The essence of budo: a practitioner's guide to understanding
the Japanese martial ways / Dave Lowry.—1st ed.
p. cm.
ISBN 978-1-59030-846-2 (pbk.: alk. paper)
1. Martial arts—Japan—Philosophy. 2. Bushido. I. Title.
GV1100.77.A2L635 2010
796.8—dc22
2010022460

Contents

v

PART THREE: REFLECTING ON THE WAY

INTRODUCTION

You can, if you want, pursue your martial art as a pleasant hobby.

You can look at your *budo* as a way to make yourself stronger, more confident, as a way to win championships, or attain status, or socialize with others who share your interest. You can use your martial arts practice as an indulgence in romanticism, pretending you are a "modern-day samurai." No one's thought to leave me in charge of how you should or shouldn't engage in your martial arts training. I'll tell you this much, though: You want to follow budo as a Way? You want to pursue a martial art as a medium through which to approach and understand life? Then there's some stuff you'd better do and some stuff you'd better know.

First, you'd better know that budo are a lot of hard work. You are reading this book. And it doesn't have any how-to pictures in it. Those two facts immediately establish that you are not the sort who just shows up at the dojo and goes through the motions, or the sort who thinks that budo is exclusively about perfecting physical technique. You understand there are other components in budo and that engaging one's intellect is far from a pointless endeavor in learning to understand the martial Ways. That's nice. And profitable for me, the writer of this book. But it's also easy to get the idea, reading books and contemplating the great mysteries of the martial Ways, that sweat, blood, and tears aren't really all that necessary. They are. In copious amounts at times. The budo are lots and lots of hard, physical work: perspiring in the dojo and being achingly numb with cold in there as well. They are about training when you don't feel like it, about being afraid, being bored, being so tired you don't think you can do one more technique. That's why, while this book can't make you stronger or technically more skilled, I've devoted the first third of it to suggestions for addressing the physical and mental aspects of the budo.

Second, you'd better understand right away that the budo are essentially, fundamentally, an expression of traditional Japanese culture and values. Yes, they have been "Westernized," to some extent, even in Japan. That isn't all bad. It is, in any event, inevitable. Institutions like budo change. They evolve. And devolve. They have, during their history, grown rich in meaning and value as human endeavors. And they have become impoverished at times, leeched of some of their profundity and energy. There was never a moment in the history of the martial arts and Ways of Japan when the budo were frozen in some ideal incarnation. There was never a "golden moment" when the martial Ways of Japan reached their summit of perfection and from which they have been in a sad decline ever since. They have ebbed and flowed throughout their existence. The addition of Western influences is only one more chapter in their story, and it isn't necessarily or even probably the definitive chapter. There is nothing inherently evil in "Westernizing" Japanese budo to some extent.

Try to strip away too much of the cultural appointments the budo intrinsically possess, however, and you will risk destroying their fundamental meaning. That means that if you want to follow the budo, you must be willing to play in a different ballpark than the ones with which most of us are familiar and in which most of us have played. Budo isn't just a more exotic form of sport or activity than the more normal ones we know. It isn't like joining a softball league. Or taking up fly fishing. It's in a different park, with different rules. If you are serious about it, you have to learn what that park is like and what those rules are. Those rules of the budo depend a great deal on tradition. For that reason, the middle third of the book deals with that subject: the traditions of the Japanese martial Ways.

Finally, if you are serious about your budo you must understand that there are influences on it, and so by extension, on you, that are not always immediately observable or obvious. Having sincerity, dedication, a willingness to exert yourself and learn: these are vital if you are going to pursue a budo seriously. You must understand that there are other elements, however, that will play a role in your maturation as a martial artist. The way you choose a teacher, the way that teacher got his own training, the attitudes in the dojo that have resonances outside it: all these are factors with which you must contend if your budo is going to be a transformative and worthwhile part of your life. If there is one area I think needs critical improvement in the budo, it is in the matter of how we question, evaluate, and explore some of the less obvious areas of our training. Most of these areas present their own challenges and some dilemmas, and in some cases it is their contemplation rather than any specific answers we might get that provide their true value. The final third of this book is given over to some of these points for reflection.

For me, these three areas—hard and well-informed physical training, understanding tradition, and contemplating the wider questions posed by a serious study of the martial Ways—are inseparable, intertwined, and equally important. Each plays a role in elevating and distinguishing the budo from many other kinds of pursuits. All have been essential for me and the many others I have known who have made these arts a part of our lives. I hope this modest collection of essays will be valuable for those *budoka* who are intent on following the same path.

Dave Lowry
Soko sho, 21 Heisei
(*Written at the first frost, 2009*)

Part One

REFINING TRAINING

1

LETTING ME WIN

YOU AND I ARE ENGAGED in an exchange of techniques. Doesn't matter what form of budo we're doing. Karate, or judo, or aikido, or kendo, or whatever. Doesn't matter the exact nature of the exchange. We can be in the midst of a free exchange of techniques—"free sparring"—or prearranged, multistep encounters of attack and response or just practicing a single technique against one another, one of us receiving and the other initiating. And you are, in whatever specific form this exercise takes, technically at least, my senior. This puts you in an interesting spot. Your experience in the art is such that you can, without much difficulty, frustrate any move I make. If you are the attacker and I am trying to meet your attack and deal with it successfully, you can, with superior timing or skill, overcome my response. If you are receiving my attack, my throw or my kick or my pinning technique, you can, in most cases, evade or overcome it. That's natural. You're technically more skilled than I am. And so what do you do? Do you use the exercise as a means of showing me just how much I don't know, never once allowing me to complete the technique? Do you use me as a kind of dummy or punching bag, throwing or hitting me again and again to get in some "practice" of your own?

No, of course not, you say. You insist that you will "let me" practice my techniques, helping me along, improving my skills. That kind of mutual cooperation is one of the hallmarks of a good dojo, you will insist. Okay. But just how much are you going to "let me" be successful? By what margin will you allow me to execute the technique? Will you just, oh, roll over and go limp and let me throw you or strike you without the slightest resistance? If not, how much resistance will you give me? Yes, you "let me win." But how, exactly, do you do that? The answer to that question is not nearly so simple as it may appear to anyone unfamiliar with the dynamics of the Japanese budo. And it illustrates an aspect of our training in the budo that can be extremely difficult to understand and properly employ. If we take this mentality to the extreme, if you "let me win" when it is your turn to be on the receiving end of a technique, you can collapse your defenses completely. Allow me to virtually do the technique without any resistance at all on your part. In essence, you become a kind of animated training dummy, allowing yourself to be completely open and not offering me any kind of defense. What do I learn from that? Not much of value. I learn to do a technique against a completely compliant opponent. Unfortunately, there aren't many of that sort of opponent I am likely to meet, either in competition or in real-life combat situations. At some level, unless I am in a fantasy world, I know that. Just as you know, as my senior in skill, that if you really turn it on, really use all your skills at defense, that you can prevent me from ever completing a successful technique against you. So you take a position somewhere between those two extremes. Your complicity in allowing me to do the technique is graduated. The first few times I am learning it, you might permit me to punch or kick at you without evading or blocking. You may allow me to throw or pin you, never locking out my movement or frustrating it. Once I have the idea, though, you will begin to turn up your defense. The better I get, the more resistance I find in you. That is the ideal relationship between a junior and senior. The senior always challenging, but not challenging so much that he discourages his junior or causes the junior to go off on a tangent, trying to use brute force or speed to gain what he should be learning through the application of technique.

Refining Training

This would be a rather simple process if only all people learned at the same rate and in the same way. Of course, we do not. Even if we did, there are other matters with which to contend in this equation of a "graduated resistance" method of learning and teaching. People, being people, bring all sorts of attitudes to the dojo. Some beginners, when you allow them to complete a technique unimpeded, will assume their success had nothing to do with your cooperation and everything to do with their amazing ability to learn and master the technique. You can almost see their egos growing. "Oh, yeah! My front kick went right to his midsection. I've got this *down!*" The face of the student in a grappling art like judo or aikido, the first time he throws another person, is often a study in the beatific. They beam. Their expression is a combination of surprise and joy. "Did I really do that?" And quickly, very quickly in many cases, that happiness turns to self-confidence—and then to a cocky sort of self-assurance that is in no way warranted. The student begins to strut a bit. You might see him a little later in class, working with another partner, and suddenly he's giving instruction, explaining, on account of his suddenly acquired expertise, just how that kick or throw is supposed to be done. After all, he just did it without any problem against a senior, right?

Other beginners in the dojo come in to training with such low self-esteem and lack of self-confidence that if they meet any resistance at all to the techniques they try they will simply quit, convinced this stuff isn't for them. Of course, as you might assume, most newcomers will fall somewhere in between on this spectrum. The point is, it is not an easy thing at all for a senior to pair off with a junior and act as a leader who can guide the junior through the basics of a technique or a training exercise. It requires sensitivity. And awareness. A senior in the dojo can never just be a training dummy that moves. He isn't *receiving* a technique when he's working on one with a junior. He is *interacting*. In one situation he may be offering only minimal resistance or evading just a little bit. In another, he has to ramp it up. His job, when he is on the receiving end of things, is to find a balance. Sometimes he must be a step behind his junior, sometimes on the same step, and most often, just a single step ahead. His actions must not be far enough above the level of the junior to make things impossible—but not so close as to make them too easy.

This kind of mentoring can be even more difficult to practice correctly when the junior begins to approach the technical level of the senior. The closer our abilities, the more challenging grows the process. You are no longer "letting me" do the technique. As I get closer and closer to you in terms of skill, you have to keep making it tougher for me. And that isn't easy. Have you ever seen a senior surprised when he's been coasting along, training with a junior, and suddenly he is hit or thrown? If not, eventually you will. It happens all the time in a good dojo. When it does, it is informative to see the results. It is also worthwhile to watch to see what the teacher, who should be overseeing things, does as well. Sometimes in these situations the senior will react with angry embarrassment. He'll come up with some admonition or explanation. "Well, yes, you got me, but you see, here's what you did wrong..." What the senior should do— what he *must* do if he is a serious budoka—is acknowledge his junior's success, or alternatively, acknowledge that he, as a senior, was not being sufficiently attentive to things. It isn't the junior's fault if the senior fails to keep a step ahead in the exchange of techniques. It is the fault of the senior. He must recognize that fault in his conduct and take it as a positive sign that he, as a senior, has had more training to get to where he needs eventually to go. If he does not do this, you should see the teacher step in, perhaps not directly but in a convincing manner nevertheless, to set the senior straight. If the teacher does not, the junior is left to wonder what's going on. If the senior behaves in a way that is not productive to the progress of the junior, that senior must be corrected. The junior is in a perilous position here, exposed. He depends upon the senior, and when he advances to a more senior role in the dojo, he will naturally use the example of the seniors before him.

"What are you doing? That's not right! The only reason you got that technique in on me is because you weren't doing what I told you to do. How can I teach you if you don't follow instructions?" The junior who hears this sort of pseudo-criticism wonders if he's really done something wrong or if the senior is just trying to cover for his own sloppiness. Usually, unless he is very immature, he sees through the senior's charade and loses confidence in the senior and perhaps in the dojo itself. As I said, it is a critical time. The teacher who allows a senior to come up with diversionary rationalizations or other stratagems to protect his own ego at the expense of the junior is going to have big, big problems, sooner or later.

The role of the teacher in these interactions is crucial. His competency in dealing with these situations, as much as any technical or teaching skills he brings to the dojo, will mean the difference between a serious dojo and what amounts to little more than a gym. The teacher is at the top of this junior-senior stair step of graduated response. Just as the seniors interact with their juniors, he interacts with everyone in the dojo. He is responsible for watching all that goes on in the dojo. Constantly he is monitoring the junior-senior relationships, watching to see that his seniors are staying out there in a technical sense, not too far but just far enough, of the juniors. And of course, there will be times, especially when working with his senior students, when he will be the one setting the pace, trying to pull them along, and giving them just enough resistance to keep them working. Following a traditional budo implies a profound sense of loyalty to a teacher and a willingness to understand that that teacher is not perfect and has flaws just like everyone else. Mine do. And one forgives these or, more properly, puts them in perspective. However, if ever I were to complete a technique against a teacher—not because I am better than him but rather because he became sloppy or inattentive—and he found some excuse, chose to excoriate me for some spurious reason to salvage his own ego, I would be out the door. This behavior is excusable in a senior. He has a teacher there to correct him. But if you are calling yourself a teacher and you abuse a student in this way, I want nothing to do with you.

Some readers may never have thought of this vital role of "graduated resistance" in the training scheme in a dojo. I hope they will. I hope they will begin to watch for it and, as they progress in the art, they will begin to employ it themselves. It is a vital part of training in the traditional dojo and a vital part in the maturation of the martial artist.

2

BASHING ABOUT

MOST READERS WILL BE FAMILIAR with *tameshiwari,* the karate practice of breaking boards, bricks, tiles, and whatever other materials might be found that seem to possess sufficient tensile strength to at least look impressive when they are assaulted. The average reader will most likely know, too, that this practice has an antecedent in *tameshigiri,* or cutting objects with the Japanese sword. Tameshigiri began as a sort of quality control check used by sword makers to evaluate their products. Swords undergoing a test of tameshigiri were fitted with special, heavy-duty grips. The targets were human bodies, either corpses of condemned criminals or the criminals themselves, hacked apart while still alive. It was a gruesome business, certainly. The point was to test the strength and durability of the blade when put to the use for which it was intended, which was, of course, slicing into human flesh efficiently.

Later on in the exercise of tameshigiri, other materials were substituted for human bodies. Bundles of tightly wrapped straw soaked in water simulated the density and resistance of a body, a sort of feudal-age version of ballistic gel. Lengths of bamboo were also used for test cutting. (Technically, by the way, cutting objects other than bodies is not tameshigiri, even though that term has become popularly used. It is *suemono-giri,* which means "to cut a fixed target.") Today, tameshigiri has a number of enthusiastic followers who use these bamboo and bound-straw targets, along with wrapped sections of *goza,* the thin straw mats of the sort you will find unrolled on the sand for a day at the beach. The clean cutting of any of these materials, by the way, is not as easy as it sounds. Legends of the sharpness of the Japanese sword are not always exaggerated. Yet even with such a keen edge, keeping a consistent *ha-suji,* or cutting angle, is tricky while swinging the sword. The sword tends to twist and jerk in one's grip when it encounters resistance. Cuts are often ragged or incomplete unless the person knows what he is doing.

Fewer readers will know of a later development in this business of testing swords: *aratameshi.* Aratameshi came about after Westerners, by threat of force as well as by the lure of trade, arrived off the coast and opened Japan from its long cultural isolation in the middle of the nineteenth century. The effects on Japan of this opening were enormous and far-reaching. Aspects of the changes wrought in Japanese society by Western ideas and technology were hinted at in the 2003 movie *The Last Samurai.* For hundreds of years, the Japanese were insulated from almost all outside influences. Their technology, their social conventions, their philosophies—all these developed independently and with virtually no competition. With the arrival of the West in their midst, for the first time, the Japanese had something new and different against which their ideas could be compared and tested. This proved to be a wonderful opportunity for artists and craftsmen, who got a vigorous infusion of new concepts and inspirations. Art from this period of Japan shows a dramatic change. However, the introduction of new ideas and new technology must have been frightening to some in Japan. They were accustomed to the status quo. The samurai, the professional warrior class of Japan, in particular was suddenly faced with military powers, techniques, arms, and strategies that were entirely foreign. Weapon makers were in a similar position. For generations, their swords and other arms were the state of the art simply because they were products of the only art there was. The sudden appearance of Western arms would have been worrisome if not actually intimidating. Was the steel of their swords, spears, and other blades really as invincible as these traditional Japanese craftsmen always believed? How would it stand up to that in Western weapons?

Probably this challenge had much to do with the introduction of aratameshi. In aratameshi, it was not the skill of the swordsman or even the workability of the sword that was "tested." Instead, the sword was simply put to abuse until it broke. The ingenuity in finding ways to mistreat a sword in these aratameshi tests was astounding. They were hammered, on the sides and back of the blade, with oak staves. The flat of the blade was slapped into a tub of water repeatedly. Deer antlers and cow horns were chopped with swords. Iron bars were hacked. Bags filled with the iron sand used in forging metal for swords were targets, slashed at repeatedly. The edge of the sword—any sword—under this kind of treatment would eventually chip, of course; the blade would sooner or later shatter. The point wasn't to see how strong or sharp the sword was. It was to see how much mistreatment it could withstand before it broke. Lesser quality blades tended to bend and warp before they snapped, but no matter. The "test" wasn't over until the weapon had been rendered useless.

I have often wondered about the mentality behind aratameshi. It never made much sense to me. It would be like using a well-made revolver as a hammer, trying to see how many nails could be pounded in with the butt of the gun before it eventually broke. Or using a fine, expensive ink pen as an ice pick, chipping away with it until the pen was smashed. Other than idle curiosity and perhaps a not altogether healthy desire to destroy an object, what's the point? The sword was not designed and developed to have its spine used as a striking point. It was not crafted to withstand percussive stress from the side of the blade. No swordsmith would ever have insisted his work was impervious, indestructible.

The point, I suspect, was, in many cases at least, a sense of inadequacy on the part of the Japanese of that period. Imagine how we might feel if, tomorrow, a spacecraft from another galaxy appeared on earth, one capable of travel faster than the speed of light, fueled by some source we couldn't even understand. We would be fascinated, one part of our nature intrigued and excited. Another part of us, however, would suddenly feel very, very inadequate. There would be a tendency in some to say, "Well, yeah, but just how good are they at . . . ?" We'd want to find something superior about our own civilization that could make us feel better about it. It would lead, maybe, to all sorts of silliness, outrageous displays and stunts of meaningless bravado. I suspect aratameshi may have, at some part of its roots, this spirit as an unconscious justification. Even if it means destroying an object, we will do so to try to prove its value—and by extension, *our* value as a people and as a culture.

Not to make too much of it, but sometimes I think we see this same attitude in martial arts today. For the great majority of it, the practical, combative applications of a fighting art are skills we may put to use once or twice in our lives, if at all. In fact, most of us will never in our lives strike another person with the intent to do harm. Police and military people are an exception, obviously. But hand-to-hand combat just isn't a part of daily life for most budoka. Sporting competitions featuring budo in some form tend to have rules that often eliminate what are supposed to be the most effective of an art's repertoire. In short, we are left with no "real" way to test the effectiveness of our arts—at least in terms of their combat value.

Movies and other depictions of martial arts portray these martial arts as lethal. Still, in that hidden part of the mind of many a budoka lies the unspoken thought: does this stuff really work? We worry sometimes that it may all be a sham, that we're like that Bedouin bad guy who's flourishing his swords in a furious display of artistry, only to have Indiana Jones pull out a six-shooter and casually blow him away. In the face of these kinds of doubts, sometimes we create fanciful "tests" of the worth of what we're doing. Whole forests have been denuded for lumber broken in karate displays. Enough ice to save the polar caps has been smashed. Every carnival sideshow test of strength and endurance has been employed, ripping phone books as a demonstration of ki power, or demonstrating one's internal power with sledge hammers smashing concrete slabs on one's chest.

In some instances, these stunts are obviously meant to get attention, either to the person or to a school or system being promoted. In some, though, I wonder if it isn't a frantic attempt to demonstrate not to others but to oneself that, yeah, this stuff really *is* worthwhile, it really does give me the special powers I want it to. I suppose there is nothing inherently wrong with these kinds of tests or this kind of motivation. But we probably ought to be doing some thinking about their overall worth. Are they a test of the tools we use, much like the smiths who tested their blades for keenness and edge? Or are they more like a frenzied display that is ultimately self-destructive, bashing away in feats that "test" power and skills that have nothing to do with budo?

3

BAKING A CAKE

IT IS A SURE BET that somewhere in your city there is a self-defense class of one sort or another being offered right now. People have been kept safe, lives saved, through lessons learned in these classes. It is amazing how many people meander through life on autopilot. They are largely oblivious to their surroundings and to the potential for danger. Self-defense classes, if they accomplish nothing other than to educate the class-takers into becoming more aware, are probably worthwhile.

On the other hand, these self-defense programs can have at least a couple of liabilities. First, they can make graduates believe they have greater combative skills than they do. Believing you are immune from danger because of talents you have acquired in a self-defense course is a setup for disaster. Good self-defense programs should not make you less fearful. They should teach you to channel your fear usefully to better detect potential dangers and to respond more effectively when meeting those threats. The second possible liability in these classes is that they often concern themselves—if you'll entertain my analogy— with mixing the icing while neglecting the baking of the cake.

Let's establish this upfront: teaching a normal person (that is, someone with the normal, socially ingrained restraints against violence) how to react effectively in a stressful situation like a fight, or even to engage successfully in a verbal confrontation that has not yet become physical, is enormously challenging.

Here is a scenario that is almost certainly being played out in some gym or dojo or community center somewhere. A teacher is grabbing a student's wrist, then showing the student how to exert a pull or jerk aimed against the thumb side of the teacher's wrist. And effortlessly, given the shape of our hand and its musculature, the grip is broken. Next, having mastered that technique, the student and the rest of the class will go on to explore other "tricks." They are taught an escape from a bear hug from behind, addressing it with a backward snap of the head to strike the attacker's face, followed by a slamming elbow into his ribs, and so on. These techniques work, to be sure. Putting confectioner's sugar in the icing will "work" as well, making the icing sweet and palatable. Learning to put sugar in the mix for icing, however, does not make you a baker.

You learn to become a cake baker by mastering certain fundamentals of this rather complex aspect of cookery. You learn how leavening agents cause a cake to rise. You learn how fats affect the texture of the cake, as well as how adding liquids will determine much about the finished cake's consistency. You learn how oven temperatures can be manipulated to make different sorts of cakes, from a light, fluffy angel food cake to a thick, dense fruitcake. You are exposed to the many different kinds of pans and forms used in baking cakes. At the outset, you must stick entirely to the rules of cake baking being taught. You master them. As you progress, you are shown shortcuts or substitutions in ingredients that make the baking more efficient and easier. You gain competency so that even in an unexpected situation—I'm short on eggs but I know I can use a little more milk to get the same result—your cakes come out as you wish. When you have learned all these fundamentals and can apply them in your cake baking without having to constantly check a recipe or your notes, you are ready to begin the next stage. Lessons now might commence in some of the finer details of cake making. Your teacher does not have to begin each session with a review of the basics. At this stage you can learn how to mix and apply the final step in creating a cake, the icing.

In a budo, the "cake" is not, as some might believe, in the *kihon,* or basics. It is not in the kata or other prearranged practices. The cake, the underlying structure that gives the budo their particular shape and taste—I know I'm stretching the metaphor more than a bit, but stay with me—is the way in which the art organizes your body and your mind. It is the comprehensive sense of the budo, and the development of a systematic way of perceiving things, based upon the central, unifying concepts of that version of the budo, that provide the cake, the "heart" of the matter.

The problem is that those enrolled in self-defense classes mistake the individual tricks they often learn there for a comprehensive skill. These tricks, individual and isolated techniques, are not that. It is like learning to make various forms of frosting and believing you know how to make a cake. It is going about things exactly backward, at least from the perspective of the martial Ways and the methods by which they have always been transmitted. The ability to make a good icing has limited use if you don't know how to make the cake on which it goes. Let's go back to that scenario I described above, of the self-defense class teacher demonstrating an escape from a wrist grab. The student can break free. But look how she is standing, flat-footed, squarely facing her opponent. What happens next? In a class, the pair might trade sides and continue practice. In reality, we know someone grabbing your wrist usually has further designs. Usually malevolent ones. Your breaking loose of the attacker's grab might mean he will proceed to launch another assault. You started out free. He seized you. You have simply returned back to the starting point of the confrontation; you have not moved into any better position.

The approach to teaching a budo correctly is to begin teaching a person how to organize his body, his posture and movement, in a coherent and systematic way. That is why you see beginners in a karate dojo moving up and down the floor repeating techniques, front kick–reverse punch and such, again and again and again. In a judo dojo, beginners will start a throw, going in just far enough to un-balance their opponent, then backing out and going in again, over and over. They look robotic. What they are really doing is training their muscles to make that kick or that throw without any conscious thought being involved, to keep their balance even when they tire. On an even more fundamental level, the budoka's mind and muscles are being shaped in a specific manner. The same goes for other basics in budo training. Kata, for instance, particularly at a beginner's level, are not about instilling technique. They are about training in coor-dinated movement, maintaining balance and body integrity while turning or shifting, about controlling all the parts: arms and legs, in ways that make sense from the point of view of that particular Way. The kata, in some aspects, anyway, are about being able to make a cake that comes out of the oven edible and tasty, without consulting a recipe or even giving the process much thought at all. The art be-comes, through time and repetition, natural and spontaneous.

A person who has a good sense of balance, who understands con-trolling his space as well as how to invade and take advantage of the space of another, can deal with a wrist grab in a dozen different ways. All those methods, however—escapes, counterlocks, joint manip-ulations—are the icing on the cake. They can change with different circumstances, just as a baker can vary the flavor of the icing, or its consistency, or the amount he may need to cover the cake before him. Learning to do this is relatively simple. (That is why, under the carefully controlled circumstances of the self-defense class, the tech-niques do indeed "work" as they do.) Acquiring the reactions and musculature and mindset necessary for implementing them at will, under unexpected conditions, as one advances in age—that is the real art.

I hasten to add that we are, if I can extend the food analogy in a different direction, comparing apples and oranges. The self-defense class is usually intended for the non–martial artist. He is not in the class to spend years and years at the task of learning a fighting art, as the karateka is. There are limitations on time that factor into what is taught in these classes and how. Someone who wants to learn to follow a simple cake recipe can be taught the technique for that particular cake in a single class. There is nothing illegitimate about that enterprise, though there should not be any assumption that the graduate of such a class is truly a baker. Further, there are serious limitations in such an undertaking. The budoka in this sense is trying to become a baker, to be able to produce, no matter what the circumstances, a dependable product. His goals are comprehensive rather than particularistic. That process is complicated, arduous. As the history of the martial Ways suggest, however, there is no better or easier way to get there.

4

DEMONSTRATIONS

DEMONSTRATIONS CAN BE AMONG the more valuable and useful tools for polishing the budoka's skills. Even if they are rehearsed—and I believe they should not be, as we'll get to in a minute—they put you as a participant under pressure. You are at the center of attention when you demonstrate. Crowds are watching. Mistakes, if they are made, are embarrassing. You are representing your art and your dojo. It isn't the sign of a big ego to want to do well in a demonstration necessarily. It is an understandable wish to present the art and your dojo in the best light possible.

There are actually two different kinds of demonstrations the budoka should be aware of. *Hono embu* is the term for demonstrations performed specifically in honor of one's ancestors in the art. Strictly speaking, hono embu take place only in the dojo or within the precincts of Shinto shrines that have some connection with the particular art. (Very strictly speaking, you might be interested to know, an art is not really officially practiced *outside* the precincts of that shrine.)

What we usually think of as a public demonstration is called, in Japanese, *shucho embu*. *Shucho* is a term from the feudal-era battle-field. The samurai of that age would ride as an individual out into the middle of the field. Standing by himself before the enemy, he would plant a flag with the crest or colors of his family or clan into the ground there, and in a loud voice announce his pedigree as a warrior. These were displays meant to impress the enemy, to warn opponents of what they were in for, and to establish one's name and reputation in the event one were killed. Those who took his life would have some idea of who the warrior was. True, the practice was not terribly effective compared to modern warfare. (And it was never the only way combat was waged in premodern Japan. Some battles at some times began this way. Others did not. No matter how they started, with formal declarations or by surprise ambush, massed warfare was complicated, frantic often, and inevitably brutal and bloody. Don't fall for romantic, modern interpretations of "samurai combat" as elegant and stylized.) But the practice sheds light on the meaning of a public demonstration of budo today. We are stepping out, placing ourselves at the center of attention, explaining who we are and what we do and then demonstrating it.

It is only my opinion, but I wish more dojo were more careful in the sites and situations where they demonstrate their art. I think in many cases, teachers or dojo leaders think initially about how a public demonstration might be of value in the short term. By that, I mean they see it as an opportunity to get the art in front of large numbers of people. They see it as a chance to expose their dojo. No doubt it is. That's why it is common to see martial arts demonstrations at shopping malls or county fairs or harvest celebrations or lots of other community events. With hundreds or even thousands of people seeing these demonstrations, it seems a good bet. Your dojo will pick up new members. It is a free advertisement, in fact.

This is a short-term look at the value of these demonstrations. Long-term, the perspective is not always so great. First, in terms of prospective, serious, potentially long-loyal members of your dojo, think about the differences in the person who seeks your dojo out versus one who has your art presented to him as a form of entertainment or a diversion. The latter might actually be motivated to show up and take a few classes. The demonstration was exciting and highlights the more dramatic aspects of your art. How long do you think he'll stay, though? He isn't going to learn to fight against three opponents simultaneously as he saw you and your group doing in the demonstration. Instead, he's learning basics, going over them again and again. It gets boring fast, and that initial interest generated by the demonstration he saw is a fire that goes out quickly. Compare him to the person who developed an interest in your budo and researched, asked around, and came to you. He's already shown the kind of initiative that is likely to have him coming back. And staying.

It is easy for me to say this. I don't have to pay the rent at the beginning of each month for a dojo. I don't depend on new students to keep the doors open as some do. I can afford to be picky and very selective about the events and circumstances under which I will demonstrate. I understand others do not have this luxury. However, while having enough students to cover the rent and utilities is important month to month, it is a poor business strategy to think entirely in such a short-term way. One must also consider the long-term effects such demonstrations have on your dojo and on your art in general. Do you want these to be taken seriously? Do you want your budo to be thought of as a serious enterprise, one undertaken by adults, by the sort of people who are going to make a lifelong commitment to it? Do you want your dojo to be thought of as a kind of entertainment center, a sort of arcade where visitors can go and have a good time and then leave when the novelty wears off? Do you want your art to be considered a sort of temporary attraction, a warm-up act for some main event? Customers going to the theater to see a martial arts movie might be entertained by your demonstration in the lobby. They might respond with a sort of "gee, that's neat—let's go get some popcorn and find seats" kind of momentary distraction. I don't want my art treated that way, however. So I do not deliberately place it in such situations.

There is a school of thought holding that public enthusiasm of budo should be meticulously planned and rehearsed. Some of these are clever, and some actually spectacular, especially when props like chairs or other objects are involved. They can look like Jackie Chan movies, with exponents kicking over a desktop to reach an attacker on the other side or jumping up to kick in two directions with both legs, using a convenient chair as a base for a handstand. An aikido demonstration might feature a dazzling display of a guy working his way through half a dozen staff-wielding opponents, tossing them with poise and ease. These demonstrations have an undeniable appeal. If not models of practicality, they nevertheless demonstrate the potential of a budo and the extraordinary suppleness, dexterity, and power that characterize it as an art.

Although such carefully plotted embu are entertaining, however, as a practitioner I am far more impressed with those that are preceded by a minimum of rehearsal or preparation. "Make four attacks with a knife. Overhand stab, underhand or horizontal slash—I don't care. Just come at me four times with the knife." This is the total "preparation" I once heard a karate teacher give a student, moments before they gave a demonstration. What happened was like a performance of improvisational jazz. The teacher was spontaneous. He had to be; he knew only that there would be four attack sequences and they would involve a knife. Even more memorable have been those demonstrations where the student is suddenly put on the spot. (These are lamentably few; teachers seem to want to be at the center of things, although it is so much more effective when they step back and either act as attackers or allow their students to do the demonstration.)

"I'm going to attack you—first with punches, then I'll switch to some kicks. Then, when I stop and bow, I'll follow with some grabs—wrist, arm, around the waist from behind. Let's see what you can do." Again, this was the extent of prefatory information given an aikido student only moments before the embu. Want to see what an art is made of? That's a very good way.

I know it is nice to see lots of synchronization, military-type precision, and drill-team sorts of demonstrations. I would encourage teachers, though, to think about having an evening in your dojo, a sort of "talent night" presentation. Invite families and friends of dojo members or others who may be interested. Just tell the students they will be expected to demonstrate. Don't tell them what. Half an hour before the demonstration, gather them and give some brief instructions: "You, perform a kata of your choosing. You and you, do a three-minute demonstration against attacks from the rear. You three, do a two-on-one self-defense demonstration. You, demonstrate this kata and have those four guys help you to demonstrate its applications. All of you have ten minutes to talk about what you're going to do among yourselves, to plan it out as best you can. Then you're on."

These won't be the best embu ever presented, I'm betting. They may not impress the crowd. They will teach those participating, however, some valuable lessons.

5

STAMINA

You do not have enough stamina.

Possibly the best lesson you can give yourself if you are a karate or kendo practitioner is to do a kata fifty times. If you are an aikidoka or a judoka, execute a throw fifty times against an opponent, then take his throw another fifty. I do not mean doing a kata or a technique fifty times with full speed, commitment, and power. (If you think you can perform a kata or a technique with these three elements all ramped up to 100 percent fifty times, you don't understand speed, commitment, and power as they apply to the budo. Either that or you are superhuman. Call me cynical, but I think the first is more likely.) No, I mean just floating along through the movements of the kata or the throw, making the stances as they should be made, moving at the correct speed but without any more force or power than you need to make the motions and get the job done. Go ahead. Try it. We'll wait. When you come back, you're going to be winded. Exhausted. While you try to get your heartbeat back down to a level that would be alarming even for a peripatetic hummingbird, you will be explaining to yourself that your inability to do this isn't really a reflection on your ability.

The martial Ways aren't a long-distance race, you'll tell yourself. Most "real" fights don't last more than about half a minute, anyway.

Explosive power is more important in fighting than slogging it out for several minutes at a time. Even professional boxers only go at it for three minutes before taking a break, you will say to yourself. Well, okay. If you can last six rounds with a boxer, even wearing headgear and overstuffed gloves and that boxer just playing around with you, I will consider the validity of that argument. I'm betting the vast majority of budoka could not do that. That is not a valid criticism of the budo or budoka, I hasten to add. Boxing is a sport that demands extraordinary stamina. To say that budo is not effective as an exercise or as a means of self-defense or that budoka are all a bunch of couch tubers because they cannot participate in a boxing match is like saying you should never strap on your cross-country skis unless you can compete in a 10K race. However, if you are serious about your martial art, you need to take a long, hard look at your stamina level.

Aerobic fitness has obvious benefits beyond what we are able to do in the dojo. The role it plays in preventing heart disease and other coronary woes is both enormous and well documented. Stamina allows us to excel to our best in budo; it is as well a fundamental means by which we can live a productive, useful, and enjoyable life. But from any persepctive, stamina does have a crucial place in our training as martial artists. It has implications beyond what we might find in sports or in a general fitness regimen.

The best definition of stamina is "the ability to maintain a sustained effort under stress." I am certainly not a physician or an exercise expert of any kind. My suggestion would be that you consult one of these. (Your sensei may be wonderfully skilled and knowledgeable about karate or judo or aikido or whatever; but he may not necessarily understand the physiological and medical mechanics of stamina, and you should not expect him to.) When you do consider the part stamina plays in your training, think of these three general areas that comprise it.

The first component of stamina is *cardiorespiratory capability*. Simply put, this is the capacity for fueling activity. How well do you use the oxygen you're breathing? How efficiently do you burn the calories you take in? There is one way to improve your cardiorespiratory capacity: you must get your heart rate up and keep it up for a period. You can run, bike, swim. Again, check with a doctor or expert to determine how long you need to keep up this exercise and how quickly you can safely work to that goal. While most budo can get one's heart rate up, the nature of our art is one of movement and stillness. There is no sustained stress placed on the body that lasts long enough to improve our stamina in this area. My suggestion of kata repetitions or continuous throwing comes close. Even so, you are much better off running or performing some other exercise that is more dependable in this regard.

The second component is *muscular strength*. Basically, this is your capacity to exert force against resistance. The air gets fairly thick and humid in the summers where I live. But it really doesn't offer enough resistance to challenge my muscular endurance by punching against it. Karateka developing the perfect punch or kick aimed against an imaginary opponent need to complement this by exerting energy against resistance. There are various ways in the dojo to do this. Loop a belt around the waist of your practice partner and have him step forward, using good form, as you hold both ends of the belt behind him. Because judo and aikido are antagonistic and involve a partner physically in contact with you and working against you, they promote this muscular strength more efficiently. Even so, probably the best course of action for you in improving your muscular strength is to inquire with your doctor or a physical therapist about a program of weight lifting. Weight lifting is a sadly overlooked tool in developing the martial artist. Some Okinawan karate systems have sophisticated tools like the *kongoken*—think of a giant, heavy iron paper clip—that can be lifted, flipped, or manipulated as a dynamic form of weight training. And the late Donn Draeger and others in Japan in the 1960s did judo a tremendous service by introducing scientific weight training to judo. Overall, however, martial artists have neglected this aspect of physical development.

The final component of increasing stamina is *muscular endurance*. Let's say you can lift two hundred pounds. That's impressive. However, what if you can do it only once? In fact, we need to be able to repeat actions against resistance. We need to increase the efficiency of the muscles we build. This is best done through addressing the first aspect of stamina we mentioned, sustained physical activity. As your muscles become capable of doing more against resistance, you need to increase the resistance and increase the duration of the activity. This is best done, obviously, through weight training. But by adding hills to your biking or running routines, you can also increase the amount of resistance.

Unfortunately, too many martial artists have uncritically fallen for the hazy notion that our arts are perfect and complete and that we don't need any complementary training not found in the art. The martial arts are not magic. They do not contain miraculous powers that will automatically increase our stamina simply as the result of regular training. In fact, just the opposite may be true. Evidence points to the reality that, as you become more skilled at an activity, you expend less and less energy doing it. A beginner karateka burns up a lot of energy and increases his heart rate substantially just moving across the floor making repetitions of side kicks. The more advanced student uses his energy more efficiently. That's good, in a way. That's our goal. But in using less energy or using it more efficiently, we also begin to compromise our stamina levels. The only way to overcome that is the same way it is accomplished in any other physical activity. Get the heart going at a rate that places it under stress. Keep it that way for a sustained period of time that will make it work more efficiently. Add resistance to continue to improve. Sorry that there isn't a shortcut for the budoka. There isn't one for anyone else.

6

ANSWERING YOUR SENSEI

"Do you know the kata Rohai?" I asked a karateka in the class I'd been invited to teach.

The karateka dipped his head and grimaced. "Well," he said, turning his outstretched palm up and down, "kinda."

I stopped the class. I had them sit. Time for a lecture. That is no way to answer a question in the dojo.

A lot of nonsense has been created regarding "dojo etiquette" in Western dojo. Most of it has come from teachers who have never been to Japan or who have had limited exposure to Japan's budo culture. Many early American martial arts teachers came from military backgrounds. They integrated a boot camp mentality into the dojo. In some dojo, it is just as likely my question would have been answered with a shouted, "Yes, SIR!" That is just as inappropriate as the diffident, namby-pamby reply the karateka made to me. So, what is the proper way to respond to your teacher in the dojo? I am not some all-knowing authority on the subject. I can, however, tell you how I was taught. More important, I can explain *why*.

First, there is of course the whole matter of "*Osu!!!*" In some karate and other budo dojo, this has become a mantra uttered during any conversational interaction with a teacher. Sensei walks onto the floor. "Osu!" yells everyone in the room. "Try harder," the sensei says.

"OSU!" roars the class. "Did you have juice with breakfast?" asks the sensei. "OSU!" the class bellows. It's silly. "Osu"—the best guess is that this word originated as a contraction for *ohayo gozaimasu,* a polite form of "good morning"—is an appropriate greeting between young, testosterone-fueled guys, a rough and masculine way to acknowledge one another within the fraternity of the dojo. It has evolved in this country as a universal reply in many dojo. Think of it the way we might use "hey!" when we see someone. Imagine how ridiculous it would sound if we shouted "hey!" in response to everything said to us. Yes, I know: there are all sorts of fanciful, supposedly profound explanations for "osu!" having to do with the kanji that can be used to write it. (The majority of these have been concocted by Japanese instructors who were embarrassed to admit they didn't have any idea what the expression meant.) The facts remain: "osu!" is not used indiscriminately in the Japanese karate or other budo dojo as it is here. "Osu" as a greeting is appropriate for young men in informal situations. To hear women or older people use it is as goofy as hearing the CEO of a corporation greet another CEO in a formal meeting with "Yo, dude!"

Much the same might be said of employing the nearest Japanese equivalent to "yes," which is *hai.* Some budoka adopt this with an almost furious enthusiasm. "Hai, Sensei!" If one is asked a direct question, this might be appropriate, although if you are a Westerner and your teacher is a Westerner, I cannot imagine why you would use a Japanese word when the English you normally use works just as well. (Then why call your teacher "sensei"? The reason is that sensei has some meaning, especially as a form of address, for which there is no good English equivalent. The same can be said for the names of many techniques or other terms we use in the dojo.)

Actually, the best way to respond to most of what a teacher says to you in the dojo is simply to do it. Do what he says. If he tells you to kick higher or step differently, don't "Osu!" or "Hai, Sensei" him. Just kick higher or step differently, as he instructs you to. When it comes to answering a direct question, there are two words that are most often appropriate: *yes* and *no.*

When I asked the karateka about knowing the kata, he thought too much. "Yes, *technically* I know it," he's thinking. "But I haven't really practiced it. I look terrible doing it. I don't want him to yell at me if I say I know it and then he asks me to do it and I look bad." This is what was going on in the mind of the karateka. It's all a waste of time. Karate and the other budo are about violent confrontation. They are forms of combat. There is a time to think and philosophize. That time isn't during training. If you are leading a group of men in battle and your commander asks you if you can lead a charge up that hill, you do not have time to reflect or cogitate. It's either "yes" or "no." Suppose you say, "Well, theoretically I think we have a good chance to take that hill if you factor in..." Do you think your commander is going to have faith in you? More important, do you think those under you will have the faith in you to make the charge? Make the decision and live with the consequences. That is a big part of what the budo are all about.

Okay, so you're that karateka and you answer "yes" when I ask about the kata and I ask you to do it. And you look terrible. You freeze halfway through. "I thought you said you could do it?" I yell at you. "I was wrong," is all you need to say. That hurts. That stings. It's embarrassing. So what? Remember all that stuff about how budo are supposed to be about getting rid of your ego and becoming more humble? Well, now you've got an opportunity to do that. You can be wrong about your ability to do the kata. That's not the same as saying you're a miserable failure as a person. This is the sort of training that allows you to see the crucial difference between having self-confidence and having a big ego.

Be honest in addressing your teacher. Get to the point. Don't equivocate. Don't treat him like a drill instructor or a guru. Don't waste his time with long, superfluous explanations. That's the best way to answer. That's the best way to train.

As I said, I'm no final arbiter of "dojo correctness." I've told you how I was shown to do it, and, as I said, I've explained the more important rationale behind it. I've told you why. If your sensei has some other explanation, you owe it to yourself to get it, and he owes it to you to give it.

7

BALANCE

THE WII FIT RECENTLY entered our home. I am of the generation that remembers when Pong seemed like the ultimate video technology, so I have not yet spent much time on the Wii Fit—other than to miss quite a few gates on the ski slalom course. Watching others in the family work out on it, however, I have one observation: this was clearly designed by the Japanese. I say that because the activities on the system place a significant emphasis on balance.

I dislike comparisons between Japanese and Western cultures that tend to stress alleged differences. Let's think less in terms of differences and more in a distinction between what is emphasized. Traditional Japanese arts and modes of physical activity often stress balance as much as they do strength or conditioning. That doesn't mean they exclude these other factors or that Western sports ignore balance. But rarely do you hear a Little Leaguer being lectured on his balance in the batter's box. Football players are encouraged to be faster and stronger; there are running drills and blocking dummies on the practice field. There aren't a lot of conditioning exercises, though, meant primarily to develop balance.

Probably the emphasis on balance in Japanese sports and arts has its roots in sumo. In sumo, you lose if any part of your body aside from the soles of your feet touches the ground. So it is a contest of balance along with strength, agility, and technique. In judo and aikido, balance is, of course, critical. We must keep our own and we must upset that of our opponents.

Think you have good balance? Stand, in a quiet room, on one leg for one minute. Should be easy enough. Now, get four or five dojomates to run in a circle around you while you try the same exercise. Chances are, you will find yourself struggling or even tottering. Outside stimulus disrupts our sense of balance. Keeping one's balance in a serene, meditative state is one thing. Combat implies a lot of movement, much of it chaotic. Keeping your balance under those conditions is considerably more challenging. And, from the perspective of budo, more important.

There are a wide range of exercises that will improve your balance. Interestingly, a number of relatively new fitness programs like Pilates and Gyrotonics have come onto the exercise scene that are centered on strengthening and improving the core muscles that give us stability. In the dojo our regular training can be directed toward the same goal. Kicking drills in some karate dojo, for example, where the target is head-high, arguably have little practical applicability. But they are excellent for increasing a wider range of motion and for developing balance. It is also worthwhile to practice kicks, at head level or as high as possible, extended out as slowly as possible, then held at full extension, then retracted just as slowly. Kicking this way gives you a sense of when and where your balance is strong and when it is threatened. In judo and aikido, it is always worthwhile to execute techniques both from the left and right sides and to take falls the same way, never favoring one over the other.

For some fun in the dojo, try a bout of "one-legged sumo." Face your partner, both of you standing on one leg. The goal is to cause the other person to lose his balance. You can play this in a number of ways: palms touching and pushing and backing off against the opponents' moves is a good variation. Or you can actually grapple, either getting a grip on one another's belt or, as you would in judo, grabbing lapels or sleeves.

The above are dynamic approaches to balance training. Much more sophisticated—and worthwhile over the long run though it takes a lot of patience—is a static exercise. Standing still. Just standing. No special stance. Just standing, legs about shoulder width apart, arms dangling at your sides. Again, while it seems easy, take the time, by yourself, to stand. Start doing a cross-check. Is there tension in your neck? Are your shoulders tight? Tuck your tailbone but avoid tensing any muscles in your hips that don't aid in that. Try to feel where your balance is. What is the smallest movement you can make without changing that balance point? Focus on the soles of your feet. The thought, in Japanese fighting arts, is that balance should be centered directly over a spot at the base of the ball of your foot. The Japanese characters that are used to describe this spot (an acupuncture point as well) mean "a gushing spring." All the muscles of your feet and ankles should be relaxed, with your weight directly over this bubbling spring. You might be surprised, concentrating on just this spot, about how much extra tension you have in your feet. It's wasted energy. If you take this standing seriously, give some introspection to what's going on in you and with your balance, you begin to see how really complex the budo can be.

As I mentioned, grappling arts focus, as a part of the regular training, on balance, both keeping it and taking it from the opponent. Serious karate practitioners will do the same. It is a major oversight—or just a matter of neglect—that karate makes so little use of off-balancing techniques. My suspicion is that this was the result of karate's late importation to mainland Japan from Okinawa. First, the Okinawan teachers who brought it were eager to show how karate differed from Japan's indigenous grappling arts, so they concentrated on its strikes. (A real mistake, since much of indigenous Okinawan combat arts contain or even feature sophisticated grappling methods.) Second, most Japanese karateka of that period had backgrounds in sumo or judo, and so they had a built-in understanding of the nature of balance in combat. Karateka should start thinking about movements in the kata that can be used to take an opponent's balance.

All budoka, while practicing the sorts of exercises we've outlined here, should eventually begin consciously trying to employ their principles in free exchanges of technique, in *kumite, randori,* and eventually in contest *shiai.* As you begin to explore your own sense of balance, and improve it, you will start to consider just how you can manipulate the balance of your opponent to make your own attacks stronger.

8

FIGHTING A CRIPPLED OPPONENT

IN JUDO COMPETITION when I was a schoolboy, I was usually the smallest and lightest. So it was a surprise to see the opponent facing me. He was frail. He walked with a slight limp, obviously some congenital condition. I was not the greatest judoka on the mat. But I was reasonably certain I could defeat this guy effortlessly. What to do? Go out and slam him? Throw him with some spectacular technique one always wishes to try but knows that in competition against a well-matched opponent it will never work? Or does one ease off? Play with, or at least go easy out of pity on, an opponent who is obviously technically inferior?

My situation was compounded by my youth. There is the adolescent urge to show off, to demonstrate one's skill publicly. Simultaneously, there is the fear of being thought a bully, of being ridiculed. "Great job. You beat a kid with a limp." The thought is that no matter how it plays, one cannot "win" in any sense of the word under these circumstances. Fortunately for me, my judo sensei had taught the art from the perspective not of competitive sport but as a martial art. They taught it as an art the techniques of which—and more to the point, the attitude necessary—were approached as if going into a real fight. What occurred to me as I bowed to my opponent was advice they had given me many times: Use what's necessary to defeat the opponent. Nothing less. Nothing more. We took grips, I moved about, trying to get a feel for his movement and his level. As soon as I felt an opening, I threw him. I did not take it for granted I would be able to do so. Nor did I attempt to perform some sort of spectacular technique. I did what it took to win. Nothing less. Nothing more.

Another way of expressing this is found in one of the maxims of Jigoro Kano, judo's founder. *Seiryoku zenyo* is usually translated as "maximum efficiency with minimum effort." Actually, this is one of the concepts that makes judo essentially and dramatically a martial art, one with more in common, in theory anyway, with battlefield combat than with the action in a sporting arena. It does not mean developing the power to defeat or destroy an opponent with the proverbial flick of the wrist or a magic finger strike. Instead, it means conserving one's energy, using it only as necessary and being able to adapt instantly, either ramping up that energy or modulating it down to a lower scale, as circumstances dictate.

A very funny practical joke I once saw involved a young karateka who'd achieved a reputation for his skills at breaking boards. He specialized in multiple breaks, with teams of four or five all surrounding him, all steadying boards. He would kick to the front, then turn and strike to the left, then pivot and punch to the right, moving in every direction, breaking the boards. At one of these impressive demonstrations, some senior dojo members managed to sneak in, alongside the pine that is normally used, a couple of boards of poplar, a very light wood. A child could have punched through them. The karateka began his *tour de force*, spinning and punching and kicking, screaming furiously. He struck the poplar boards with a furious knife-hand blow—and went right through them, losing his balance and crashing into the guys holding the wood. He used maximum effort—with efficiency that did far more than what was needed.

Moderating power is a valuable skill for the martial artist. There is a reason for this. Energy is always the most precious commodity, in one way or another, in a combative situation. Use it carelessly or with little sense of how it is best conserved and you are soon out of it.

Just for fun, I have often been tempted to compile a video collection of all the cinematic examples we see of "sword-twirling." You know, the movie scenes where combatants draw close together, preparing to fight, and one or both twirl their swords. The guys spin them like their swords are batons. Why would anyone outside a movie do this? What does sword-twirling do? It makes one vulnerable to a sudden attack. It creates the possibility of dropping the weapon. More to the point, spinning a sword wastes energy, however slight. In battles throughout history, men have expressed their nervousness, cleaning or checking their weapons, fussing about, stewing and fretting. They can actually exhaust themselves this way before the battle begins. True, sometimes ferocious displays, like spastically twirling *nunchaku* flails, a la Bruce Lee, or going through weird, pseudo–kung-fu gyrations, may intimidate an opponent. Mostly, though, they just bleed off vital energy for the fight ahead. I know sword-twirling is nothing more than a theatrical stunt, something designed to look cool. It illustrates, though, a good example of a waste of energy. It is energy not directed at the necessities of combat: combat requires drawing close enough to an opponent to hit him, and hit him accurately, and hit him with the force necessary to get the job done—but not being wasteful of energy in accomplishing any of that.

It is very worthwhile for the martial artist to watch predators in their hunt for prey. Predators are models of efficiency. Tigers do not roar or jump about before or while making a kill. They do only what they need to do. Lions, chasing after a herd of wildebeest that get too much of a start on them, will not pursue quarry forever. You can almost see the lions calculating, figuring how much energy output is worth the possible reward. Effective combat is much the same. Good combative systems tend to be extraordinary studies in efficiency.

We must, it is important to note, distinguish between efficiency in combat (or in the sporting arena with those combative arts that include such) and good training. In training, we will often try to go in the opposite direction, using as much energy as possible. Where one strike would be sufficient, we will repeat it dozens or hundreds of times. We make our stances lower in practice than we would in a real encounter, to strengthen muscles and improve balance. We exaggerate many of the actions of combat deliberately. The same is true in kata and or kata-like sequences. You respond to a punch at your face with a block meant to injure the opponent's striking arm or hand, follow that with a joint lock, a takedown, then a stomp. You practice such exaggerated responses because they afford you a greater range of options in a real situation and because you train with the possibility that your first or even second or third counter will not do the trick. Tiger cubs learning to hunt begin by stalking one another and engaging in protracted wrestling bouts. They are doing the same thing, learning a variety of responses that will be useful later. Significantly, as young animals, they are also burning off the excess energies of youth. It is in the mature adult, the tiger looking for a real kill, that we see real efficiency emerge.

Among the most common errors beginner martial artists make is in using too much power. Consciously or not, beginners will go full force when learning a movement or technique. It is perhaps natural. But it is a mistake. Think of learning to play a piano. Striking the keys harder, trying to make the music faster—these don't do much good. They are actually counterproductive. In budo, power comes after one has learned correct form, distancing, and timing. That isn't because power isn't important. It is because power is the most difficult of all these to manage, to conserve and use effectively. Too little and you don't get the job done. Too much—and this is what the serious martial artist needs to think about—and you waste energy. That is not something you can afford to do.

9

FOCUS

IT WAS A DOCUMENTARY, a behind-the-scenes look at the stunt team trained and led by the actor Jackie Chan. Chan, of course, is a minor movie phenomenon; his action films, liberally seasoned with comedy, are staples for millions of his fans. Chan has succeeded so well, in part, because both in his real life and in his film roles, he never seems to take himself too seriously. He's affable; invariably, Chan makes himself the butt of jokes and is never afraid to look a little silly. It is obvious, though, that he takes the choreography of his fight scenes very seriously. Most of the innovative techniques and stunts we have seen in "martial arts"–type action movies over the past two decades can be traced directly to the genius and expertise of Chan.

In this documentary, a stuntman was being coached in a complex fight sequence with Chan. He was not a member of Chan's team. He was having trouble with the sequence. Chan, a hard taskmaster apparently, went over the moves a couple of times with the stuntman, who continued to struggle. He was clearly flummoxed. A couple of Chan's team members who were also in the filmed scene began telling him what to do. He looked up at first one, then the other, bewildered. At that moment I thought, "This guy isn't a serious martial artist."

Of course, the guy might not claim to be serious about martial arts. He may well be simply a stuntman who wishes to incorporate a realistic (more or less) kind of combat art technique into his repertoire. So I am not judging him. Instead, my comment is that his reaction to that situation is one the serious martial artist ought to consider.

If we know anything at all about combat or violent situations (and fortunately, like most of you, I don't know much in terms of firsthand experience), we have learned that perceptions in these situations can radically change. Under the duress of fighting, psychologists tell us, our perception and our ability to process what we see, hear, and feel undergo all sorts of distortions. The barrel of that handgun pointed at us seems to loom larger than the end of a cannon. Or perhaps we focus on a freckle on the attacker's face, able to suddenly see it as if through a microscope. We become fixated on small details and lose the larger picture. Alternately, we may be unable to process any details at all. Merely pulling our hands out of our pockets may be more challenging, under direct stress, than solving a complex math problem. In the threat of immediate danger, some of those who have survived explain that time seems to move in slow motion. We have no clear memory of simple things: How many shots were fired? What was the color of the shirt the man had on who lunged at us with a knife?

Doubtless there are psychological and physiological explanations for these phenomena. Big parts of our normal thinking processes may shut down in order to more fully activate other processes more directly linked to survival. It was not so long ago, evolutionarily speaking, when we as a species were prey as much as predator. Our senses developed in ways that would maximize our chances for survival against a mortal threat. An unarmed man against a saber-toothed tiger would have stood little chance if he decided to stand and fight the cat. We survived—if we did—by getting away quickly. Even with primitive weapons, we were at an extreme disadvantage. As weapons became more sophisticated, the odds improved in our favor. Technically, we were gaining an edge. Our brains, though, were still wired more efficiently to flee. This led to a dissonance. Our reliance on weapons and strategies was telling us to do one thing. The limbic part of our brain, however, the part of our nature we'd brought with us from earlier times, was telling us to get running.

This dichotomy, between fighting and fleeing, is at the heart of all combat systems, in one way or another. It is relatively easy to teach a healthy human in good condition how to fight, from a purely technical perspective. Teaching him to be *willing* to fight, however, is another story entirely. We have a lot of conflicting impulses under stress. The matter of being unable to focus properly is one of them. The Japanese budo, like all combat systems, address the problem, in a variety of ways. When you see the suffix *-shin*, or "-mind," in budo terminology, it is often a reference to the attitude we carry into a stressful situation. *Isshin*, for instance, is "one mind" or a "unified mind," undistracted by anything other than the matter at hand. *Zan-shin* refers to the ability to stay alert, with a relaxed readiness at the end of a fight, to be aware of what might happen next. *Jiki-shin* can be written with characters that mean a "direct mind," in which no stray thought or emotion intrudes and the person is able to respond without any mental hindrance. These are all attempts to codify a desired combative behavior.

In the case of the stuntman in the Jackie Chan movie, his attention was distracted, divided, scattered. Probably most of you have heard of the analogy of *suigetsu*, or "the moon on the water." If the water is perfectly calm, it reflects the image of the moon without any distortion. Splash the water just a bit, though, and the reflection of the moon shatters into thousands of shards. The stuntman's mind was like that. He was listening to the actor. He was also distracted by advice and instruction being shouted at him by others on the set. It was a moment when he should have continued to look directly at Chan, raised his hands to quiet the others, and spoken in a quiet but firm voice. "Who is in charge here? Who should I listen to? Are you the boss, Mr. Chan? If so, you tell me what to do. If it's one of these other guys, tell me who it is and I will listen exclusively to him."

Now of course, in this situation, just as in any stressful situation, we cannot focus entirely on one person or one thing. It might be important for me to remember the color of the shirt of the guy who's coming at me with a knife. If I get away, that will be useful to the police in tracking him down. But I'd also better be considering possible ways of exiting or possible means of defending myself as well. If you were the stuntman we're discussing, you cannot completely tune out the others who are giving advice and instruction. You have to be aware of them, just as you have to be aware of more than one aspect in a dangerous situation. But you must compartmentalize them. You have to put them in the correct perspective. And you must be able to readjust instantly. If the actor tells you that the guy there on your left is the one who's in charge of the fight sequence in this movie, then you must make him the focus of your attention.

Focusing our attention in the circumstances of a threat does not mean we shine a laser light on one facet of the situation and ignore everything else. It means we direct the main part of our energy in one place, while being aware of whatever else is going on. Learning this attitude has reverberations far beyond training. When you go to the dojo, you cannot entirely forget you have responsibilities elsewhere in your life. They must be a part of your consciousness. Simultaneously, you have to place them in the correct perspective for the moment, concentrating on your training while you are training and not being distracted. Easy to say. As we can see in the case of that bewildered stuntman, though, it is not at all easy to do.

10

I'M READY

It was one of those movies—there must be dozens—where the young, enthusiastic new teacher confronts a classroom rowdy with loutish students who seem like junior criminals but who are, underneath the surface, really just a bunch of lovable, bright kids who merely need a chance and a firm hand to polish them into happy, productive beacons of light for the future. These kids must live exclusively in Hollywood—everywhere else young thugs tend to be just that: young thugs. Anyway, the ambitious teacher, who was, in this case, a former Marine, jumps right in and shows she's going to be something different in their lives. In one scene, a boy advances threateningly, catching her off guard. When she finally sees him, she instantly leaps into "combat mode," taking a stance, her hands cocked like swords. It's supposed to show, I guess, that she's ready for a fight.

I think in real life, a guy twice the size of the diminutive teacher who was faced with such a stance would probably be deterred in his attack mostly because he'd be laughing so hard he couldn't continue on. In real life, taking a stance in the face of a threat? Uh, not such a good idea.

Supposedly "combat ready" stances have a long tradition in many fighting arts. In the West, ritual played a big role in formal fighting.

We have all seen the fists turned and raised, making small circles in the air, the "putting up your dukes" that preceded boxing bouts of the nineteenth century. Fencing duels included salutes to the opponent and the blade held in a specific position that commenced the fight. The key here is that these are formal bouts. They may have been undertaken, in the case of fencing duels, with bloody and deadly intent. Nevertheless, they were ritualized considerably. In the case of most Japanese budo, the assumption is not that you are going into a formal contest but rather that you have been unexpectedly attacked. You go instantly from a relaxed air into combat mode. (The notable exception would be contests conducted in premodern Okinawa, between karateka who might have been representing their village or their karate system.)

If you have time to take a stance, you don't need a stance. You have other needs. A fight that allows you the opportunity to adopt a stance is one that never should have reached that point. Sure, I know all that stuff about running away from a fight. We both know that isn't always possible. What is possible, when a confrontation begins to escalate, is to take a stance, figuratively instead of physically, that starts moving things in your direction. An example: a guy leaps from his car just as you're parking yours. "You cut me off back there!" He's screaming, frothing. You can take your fighting stance and get ready for a fight. This guy is already in a barely controlled rage. What's it going to do for you to demonstrate you'd be happy to get physical as well? You are just escalating the situation and not particularly to your advantage, unless you think your display will cause him to back down. And if he doesn't, your stance just put you in a corner. It closed off alternatives. Consider this alternative, for example: Instead of taking an obvious stance, you scream right back. "I know! I am so freaking stupid! I am the world's worst driver, I swear!" You're screaming at the same level he was. You slam your palm onto your car's hood. "I can't believe how dumb I am!" If he continues to scream, you do the same, with the same intensity. Of course, your rage is an act. You look like you're out of control. But you've got your balance; you're positioning yourself so he doesn't get too close. You are keeping your hands loose and open, your elbows close to your sides. You are in a position to punch or grapple if you need to. You just don't look like it. Your "fighting stance" is nothing *overtly* of the sort.

What you are doing, obviously, is a little confusing to your assailant. He's expecting you to defend yourself, to argue or to try to explain that you weren't even aware of cutting him off. In a sense, you *are* taking a stance. You are already engaged in the confrontation. You are leading him, throwing him off balance. You are actively engaged in the situation. You are just not being obvious about it, as you would be with a stance.

Think of the potential problems in taking a physical stance when a confrontation is imminent. First, if your opponent is the sort who enjoys violence, your aggressive stance (and it is aggressive, even if you think of it as defensive) is virtually an invitation. He's all too happy to escalate in his response. Second, you are giving your opponent information. While he may not recognize the system, he'll know you have some experience in a martial art–type system. If he is a predator type, he will also instinctively spot any weakness in your stance. This is true for any fighting art, of course. A lot of boxers have found themselves writhing in pain on the ground with a knee dislocated by a savvy street fighter while the boxer was still taking his stance. Wrestlers who hunch over and raise their arms in a hugging motion have been clocked with a punch before they can close with an opponent.

The serious budoka needs to give a lot of thought and training to "stances" that are not physical postures so much as they are attitudes or strategies that employ the mental and strategic aspects of combat as well. A successful stance in this context is one in which a fight is either avoided or, if it does become physical, is entered with you already at an advantage. It has little to do with posture, with an outward show of strength or a display of intent. It has everything to do with what, in a purely combative sense, makes budo a martial art.

11

MARTIAL ARTS ETIQUETTE
(*BUDO SAHO*)

IT WAS BACK in the old days, from the perspective of most readers here—in the sixties, when judo matches were won with either a full or half point, or they were lost by the same. There were no fractional "advantages" in the scoring system of competitive judo as it exists today. Senior matches lasted five minutes. That's a long time when you're trying every technique in your repertoire and encountering a few you haven't seen yet from the other guy. Which is exactly what was happening with the two contestants we were all watching from our places at the side of the mat. I could hear their gasps as they tried to control their breathing. Mori, a young collegiate *nisei* who'd spent two years in Japan during high school, was an excellent judoka. He was fast and clean and poised. Jackson, the other contestant, was not quite up to Mori's skill level overall. But he was a clever strategist. He had been using his weight advantage to avoid being thrown. It was a stalemate. Then, when it looked like the match was going to end in a draw, Mori managed an awkward, not-quite-there foot sweep. It was a lunging attack, its force blunted by fatigue. Still, it got a response. Jackson collapsed, partly a fall, partly a stumble.

"*Waza ari!*" the referee snapped. A half point.

Mori stepped back. He took a deep breath. Then he leaned over Jackson, who still sat on the mat, to give him a hand up and help him to his feet. Jackson took the offered hand, and just when he was halfway up from the mat, still depending on Mori's grip, Mori's foot snaked out. Jackson, totally unbalanced, went down. Hard.

"*Ippon!*" A full point.

As I said, this was back in the sixties. It was a period when audiences at martial arts contests did not find it necessary to howl and scream to show their enthusiasm. It was a time when a lot of audience members knew and appreciated the difference between a sport and a martial art. Usually, though, there was some applause after a good match. At the announcement of Mori's win, though, there was an uncomfortable silence. People in the stands avoided looking at one another, and there was some squirming in the seats. Clearly Mori had won. It was an excellent example of *de-ashi barai,* an advancing foot sweep. But still . . . As one judoka said quietly in the dressing room afterward, "It just wasn't fair fighting."

Our country has been around for more than a couple of centuries now. As Americans, we are all fairly well established as inhabitants of the New World. It's obvious, however, that we in America still have a lot in common with the parent culture of the Old World. Along with the French, the Spanish, Italians, and others, we share similar linguistic roots. Our ideas about beauty and art spring principally from Europe, as do the basic forms of our literature. For the most part, in everything from cooking to economic theory, we need not look too far before we can find a similar comparison in the institutions of our European cousins. On a more fundamental level, even though they are foreign countries and cultures, the philosophies and social concepts of Europe are readily understandable to Americans. You may know nothing of their origins, but the stories of King Arthur and Beowulf probably seemed familiar the first time you read them simply because the actions and motivations of the characters were inspired essentially from the same code followed by our own cowboys and frontiersmen. Likewise, we can comprehend ideas such as the eighteenth-century struggle for French independence because we have our own revolution with which to compare it. Liberty, equality, and fraternity are common ideals in Western civilization. It doesn't matter whether they were formulated at Valley Forge or at the Bastille.

Just as certain conduct codes and mores and motivations appear universal, so do some "rules." In Birmingham, whether it's the one in England or the one in Alabama, we know there is something fundamentally wrong about endangering an innocent damsel. In a suit of armor or in chaps, a man doesn't hit an enemy when he's down. He treats others, and expects to be treated, as an equal; respects, yet healthily questions, authority; believes firmly in something ill defined but always understood as "fair play."

These similarities make it comparatively easy for us to deal with most foreigners who share a common culture with ours, either in making treaties or war with them, or in simply trying to follow the plots of their books and plays. Understanding foreign ways would be uncomplicated, to say the least, if we could always depend on such comparisons. Those, though, who take an interest in Asian, specifically Japanese, culture and traditions, are soon frustrated by the inadequacies or inaccuracies of comparisons. They find, for instance, that the damsels of feudal Japan, far from being idealized objects of romantic desire, were often ignored and neglected by the "courtly" samurai. Just as often, women in that age and place were political equals to any man, viciously capable in plotting, manipulating, and directing the political forces of their clans. Instead of the largely successful heroics of Europe's knightly tales, Japanese legends abound with noble *bushi* who *failed* in their undertakings, slitting open their bellies rather than living happily ever after. (Yes, we have failed heroes as well, from King Arthur to that steel-drivin' man John Henry. But their deaths are usually moral tales about the dangers of hubris rather than the stuff of folk heroics.) In place of the geometric symmetry of a Western garden, with its neat hedges and flowering rows of horticultural obedience, the Japanese gardener seems to take a delight in training his plants to appear wild and untended. And so it goes, getting more and more confusing.

The thoughtful scholar of Japanese tradition will soon realize that comparisons to Western cultures are limiting in understanding Eastern ways. Other less careful types will plunge ahead, determined to interpret different customs solely through the lens of their own history and experience. They can drive you nuts. They are the kind who cannot be dissuaded from the notion that geisha, for instance, are the Japanese equivalent of prostitutes. Never mind that prostitutes have always existed in Japan separate from the geisha. To these people, women who entertain men professionally are prostitutes and that's the end of it. They are incapable of seeing any distinction. Similarly, if God is worshipped in Christianity, then Buddha must be the central object of veneration among Buddhists. Try to point out to them that it isn't quite the same, and they will turn you off. They insist on interpreting all through their own culture.

To correct this kind of errant thought as it relates to Japanese traditions would require a lengthy explication of Japanese culture that is hardly within the limits of our subject here. Much narrower in scope, what we are trying to do is to gain a more complete understanding of some traditional, premodern Japanese ethics as they relate to the budo. Notice I qualified that last sentence twice. The words "traditional" and "premodern" deserve repeating here, not because I'm being paid by the word to write this but because the martial Ways are not entirely a product of the modern Japan in which they were first formalized. So naturally they do not always conform to the prevailing attitudes and behaviors there or here. They have, within them, some ethics and attitudes that evolved and were practiced in a time when feudal concepts, the stuff we have sometimes called, for lack of a better word, "bushido," were in flower. In short, the budo may have become sports or spiritual Ways. They may focus entirely on these goals or these may be by-products of their training. And it is true that the modern budo have adopted a number of markedly Western concepts within their practice and pedagogy. In some ways, in fact, karate-do and judo may be more Western than "traditionally Japanese" in their overall sensibilities. However, if they are real budo, they will have within their structure some remnants, at least, of the mentality of the battlefield and the centuries-long civil war of ancient Japan.

Jigoro Kano (1860–1938) was thoroughly a man of his time: international, cosmopolitan in his outlook. Reading what he wrote about education as well as about judo, one is constantly reminded of just how modern and Western he was. Gichin Funakoshi (1868–1957), Morihei Ueshiba (1883–1969), and other budo luminaries may have been less so, although doubtless modern thinking influenced each. Their budo reflect this. All of these individuals, however, had been raised in a Japan much closer in many ways to the sixteenth than to the twentieth century. Even if they had eventually tried to expunge traditional values from their Ways (and to some extent they did), it would have been impossible.

The origins of the samurai as a separate, recognizable class are debatable among historians. They coalesced as a fighting class under the shogun Minamoto Yoritomo. The ethical systems surrounding their class began to evolve long before that. What we now think of as the "code" of bushido, a specific set of moral and social constructs that supposedly guided the samurai class, was not really thought of in such a distinct way in Japan until the early twentieth century, when a writer and social critic, Inazo Nitobe, wrote a book extolling the virtues of the noble samurai. Originally published in 1905, the work was intended for Western readers and presented myths, legends, and history as examples of the values of the Japanese warrior class. Critics correctly observe that a lot of Nitobe's book, *Bushido: The Soul of Japan,* is a romantic, almost absurdly idealized treatment of the warrior caste. In reality, for every example of exemplary conduct by the samurai, one could find as many exceptions. "Bushido" as a values system is more an abstract concept—a very abstract one at that. In fact, it is well described in the same way that the subjects of the movie *Pirates of the Caribbean* drolly note of their own supposedly clear and inviolable "code"—that it is "more of a guideline" than anything else. As a philosophy, it was used to teach virtue and kindness to others; it was used just as effectively to rationalize murder and ruthlessness. So employing bushido as a yardstick by which to measure the behavior of the samurai of old or the modern-day budoka is largely impossible. Efforts to do so are invariably misleading. We can read the markings on that stick too many different ways for it to be useful as a way of evaluating actions or attitudes. Instead, it might be more beneficial to use the measure of *saho.*

Saho, most simply put, means "conduct." At the remove of several centuries and a political and social climate so distant from our own, it is tough for us to judge the motivations of the samurai. We can, however, look at their conduct. The same can be said for modern budoka. Many people today are geared to judge by the evidence of the end product. Conduct—the way we reach that end—is not always given a lot of consideration. Yet within the context of the Japanese budo, by elevating the status and importance of conduct, or saho, we gain a different, potentially useful, perspective. The ends are largely secondary to the means, or the conduct by which we reach those ends. This was especially important in a culture like old Japan's, where the weight of philosophical and religious thought was balanced toward the notion that winning, losing, profit, or poverty were matters determined by fate. Mankind had little control over the vicissitudes of life. What he *could* control in the face of prosperity or adversity was his saho, his conduct in the face of what fate offered.

Think of it this way: in our world we often judge individuals by the "fruits of their labor." We are willing to forgive a multitude of faults if the fruit is of sufficient abundance and sweetness. Young people can idolize and try to emulate a pop music star, in spite of the star's well-known tendencies toward reckless behavior or drug abuse, because they admire the end result he produces: enjoyable music and an opulent lifestyle. Even though she lived a life of remarkable piety, India's Mother Teresa has been applauded not for her religious devotion but because the end result of her devotion, helping India's poor and sick, has been so successful. Looking at the social and political history of Japan, we find numerous examples of "heroes" whose deeds are considered heroic even today, even though they ultimately failed at their endeavors. Kusunoki Masashige and his brother Masasue immolated one another with their swords after losing the battle at Minatogawa and putting their emperor, Go-Daigo in jeopardy in the fourteenth century. Masatsura, the son of Masashige, also committed ritual suicide after losing a battle against the Ashikaga forces. All three of these men were considered role models of sorts, not because of any success but because of their conduct under difficult circumstances. (Ivan Morris's book *The Nobility of Failure* is entirely devoted to this phenomenon among the military class of Japan.) They were admired not for what they did or didn't do, but because of their saho, their conduct and sense of decorum.

One might be tempted to say that saho is really just a Japanese way of expressing the very Western words of the sportswriter Grantland Rice: that it's not whether you win or lose but "how you play the game." You might be tempted to say that. But don't. You will have made the error we just discussed, of making impulsive comparisons. While there is something to that parallel, it is vital to bear in mind that the game and the rules by which it is played are vastly different in the budo than they are in Western sports. When a boxer sees his opponent tripped or knocked down, he steps back, waiting for the referee to make sure the man is all right and able to stand again. That is natural, since boxing is a sport and both participants, even though they may look as though they wish to commit mayhem with their fists, are actually trying to score points against one another. They are trying to win a contest. The two combatants I spoke of earlier, Mori and Jackson, were involved in a budo contest. Winning is important there also. But the primary goal in a budo *shiai* is one of self-improvement of a spiritual and physical nature. Second, contestants in shiai strive to overcome an opponent by using the techniques of their art. If Mori refused to exploit the opportunity presented by Jackson's inattention, he would have been ignoring a basic precept of judo—that of drawing an opponent off-balance, then attacking— and he would have done a disservice to Jackson by allowing a sloppy habit or gesture to go unchecked. Throwing Jackson, Mori showed that he was alert and skillful and was treating judo as a fighting art: treating his opponent, within the rules and traditions of budo, as an enemy. Jackson, we can imagine, learned dramatically and conclusively never to abandon his guard or forget that judo is a Way based upon a fighting, martial discipline. Victory or defeat was of minor importance in the lesson taught and learned that day. Both judoka experienced the moment as an exercise for improving saho.

From the beginnings of organized budo shiai, the concept of saho has been a determining factor in the establishment of its rules. I would argue, in fact, that whenever saho has *not* been a determining factor, the quality of the contests, and more important the quality of the budo, have suffered. "Traditionalists" in karate-do, for example, tend to oppose the use of protective equipment in bouts of free-sparring or contests. Like-minded judoka are critical of the institution of fractional points being allotted in scoring and of the stalling tactics that often follow as the person who has such an advantage seeks to run out the clock by becoming entirely defensive. The karateka's and judoka's rationale for these objections are fundamentally based not on the idea that these additions to the contest scene are modern or innovative but because they are contrary to the cultivation of saho.

The stresses of a contest expose a martial artist to many of the mental and physical stresses he experiences in everyday life. They give him an opportunity to develop to the fullest a sense of control over his conduct. Years ago, when judo was still practiced primarily in this country by those of Japanese ancestry or those who had some exposure to Japanese culture, tournaments were often designed with this attention to saho in mind. When I began judo in the late 1960s, a popular kind of tournament was *kachi-toru* or *kachi-nuki* (to "win through successive victories" or to "win or be left out"). They worked like this:

Contestants lined up by rank and experience. At the head of the line would be the senior black belts. At the other end were the white belts, those with the least experience. Starting from that end, the least experienced white belt and the next least experienced faced one another for the opening match. The loser of that contest sat back down. The winner immediately took on the next person in the line. He continued fighting until he was defeated. Then he sat to let the victor continue. Among the lower ranks, winners seldom lasted through more than two or three matches before they were beaten, either by another, better opponent or by their own exhaustion. (I speak from a lot of experience in that area.) But in the brown- and black-belt levels, conditioning and the ability to execute technique was often at its peak. A good and lucky judoka might go through four or five competitors before he faced one who could put him away.

Kachi-toru tournaments might seem unfair. They were. So is life. That's one of the lessons we took from it. Still, if you think about the concept, you'll see a lot of reasons why kachi-toru shiai would have some interesting elements. True, the fellow who'd just won a couple of matches would be winded and puffing for breath, and he'd be facing a new challenger who was rested. But remember: the winner was up and moving about, warm and loose. The guy he was facing had just gotten up from *seiza,* sitting on his bent knees. Those competitors waiting to fight didn't have the luxury of standing up or stretching or being "on deck." Often, some of the senior black belts had to go directly into a match when they were cold and stiff and experiencing the stabbing needles of *shibireru,* the term that describes legs gone completely to sleep from sitting in seiza for a long time. I saw a lot of those seniors thrown by lesser-skilled opponents before the senior could even get any feeling back in his legs. (Our teachers often reminded us that this is pretty much what real combat is like. Sitting around, waiting, in cramped, uncomfortable positions, and suddenly being forced into full-on action. The same is true for daily situations that might require an instant response. You don't get to warm up to prepare for a mugging or an assault.)

From another perspective, the "last man standing" was indeed the "champion." Didn't do to get too excited about that, however. If you won the last match, in some likelihood you had beaten a guy who had just faced and beaten three or four before you. What it meant was that the whole idea of "winner" got changed. One judoka might have won. But everyone was talking about the brown belt who beat six opponents in a row before he was defeated. The emphasis was not on the end result. The goal of such shiai was not to produce champions. Instead, it was designed to allow everyone involved to conduct himself or herself in a manner that displayed, under difficult circumstances, the kind of conduct that would make one successful in a real encounter or in life in general. The goal was not expressly the development of saho, true. But that was an inevitable byproduct.

Viewed from this angle, where personal behavior and the constant maintenance of a strong spirit are considered more relevant attributes than the more measurable qualities of success or failure, the ethics of the budo should become more explicable. Further, you should recognize that the traditional martial Ways have no obligation to conform to a foreign (from their perspective) sense of chivalry or fair play just because some people from another culture (ours) wish to take up those Ways.

The childish tantrums we see in professional sports like tennis might be tolerated in a modern setting. But in the Japanese budo, those antics are in utter opposition to the importance of saho. If a newcomer thinks he can indulge in them, he will very quickly find himself among others like him, those who dabble in martial Ways, excluded from serious practitioners who would never allow such behavior. Many years ago, I saw Hamilton Miyazaki, a teenage judoka friend of mine, win a contest with an excellent, clean hip throw. The referee raised his arm and shouted "*Ippon!*" to announce the full point. In exultation, the judoka pumped his fist. "*Hansoku-gachi!*" the referee shouted just as loudly. A loss by forfeit. Miyazaki wasn't smart enough to know what he'd done wrong. He *was* smart enough to know you didn't argue with a referee. He understood enough about saho to realize that. So he sat down without a word. The referee came over. Save the celebrations for later, he told Miyazaki. Lose your concentration and congratulate yourself like that out on a battlefield or in a real fight, and it could be enough to get you killed. Miyazaki nodded. He didn't like it. But he nodded anyway. At another shiai, I saw two judoka go to the ground, grappling. They weren't getting anywhere, neither with a good advantage, and so, following the rules of judo competition, the referee separated them and had them stand and go back to their starting positions. One judoka turned his back and walked back to his mark. Again, instantly the referee called the match for his opponent. The reason? Simple. Had he been in a combat situation, turning his back on an opponent was a serious, potentially lethal gap in his awareness. A gap in his saho.

Well, you are making too much of all this, might be the argument. The *shiaijo,* the contest area, is decidedly *not* a battlefield. A contest, no matter what the intent, no matter how serious the participation, is worlds away from a real situation where one's well-being or even one's life is on the line. It is a bit precious and pretentious to be treating an opponent in a judo or karate tournament as a mortal enemy. That is certainly true. We are not talking about the actual application of combat here, though. We are trying to reinforce an ethos, a state of mind that, while not engaged in a life-and-death struggle, emerges with a sense of that spirit. If you want to see budo saho, a perfect place to begin is in watching sumo. *Sumotori,* during a referee-called break in the action, do not turn their backs on one another. They do not lose their focus. They do not pump their fists or jump around when they win. They are relaxed before and after the action of a bout. But they are never slack in their attention. Their saho, their sense of propriety and decorum, isn't one of pomposity or strutting machismo. It's a kind of quiet awareness, a sober, steady bearing. Like the budo today, sumo is not a life-and-death struggle. Watch carefully the behavior of the sumotori, however, and you will see sumo isn't just a sport, either. Much of that distinction emerges in saho.

It is true that the values of the budo transcend culture. The Japanese don't "own" budo. They do not have an exclusive insight into it.

It is equally true, though, that the values of the budo are based upon tenets of a specific culture. Those for whom this is unimportant will never grasp the nature of the martial Ways. Since the ethical precepts of the budo and its ethos as well are so different from many of the prevalent attitudes we have in the West and in the modern world in general, they present a real challenge to the person who is able to overcome some of his own prejudices and expectations to try to understand budo on its own terms. Not everyone can. During my college days, I knew one fellow who could have turned himself into a fine judoka, but he could not get around his disbelief that women in the budo are treated equally to men. He refused to take seriously the female judoka we had in the dojo, in spite of the fact that some of them were better, much better, technically, than he was. While he was trying to waltz them gingerly about the mats, they were sacking him right and left. (I hasten to add that it would have made no difference if he had been better than the women. It was not his competitive record that mattered; it was the way he treated the women in training.)

Others cannot accept the concept that size is not of the paramount importance to which they attach it. Some, being large, constantly rely on their bulk, never really polishing their technique; others, being small and slight, avoid serious training altogether. Still others, the most pitiable, I think, believe traditional budo can be bent and molded to fit current attitudes or behaviors. Their interpretations are varied in form, but similar always in depth—or more accurately, in their lack of depth. Whether they mistake saho for machismo or a militant feminist ideology or with a starry-eyed "cosmic consciousness," in every case they are missing the point of saho's value and worth.

Let's be clear: traditional values espoused by the warrior class of Japan are not universally superior to any others. And notice I said "espoused." The samurai were capable of treachery, of ruthless calculation, of exploitation and obscene ambition. Sure, some of them went to their deaths with noble mien, serene in dying by having lived according to their perceptions of saho. Others went out screaming and scrambling, or sniveling and lying, in an attempt to stay alive for one more breath. No matter how corrupt or greedy modern politicians may be, there is not one of them alive today who could hold a candle to the megawatt mendacity of Oda Nobunaga or Hideyoshi Toyotomi. My point is not that the ethics and values of feudal Japan are a moral lighthouse in a dark and stormy sea. (Although I do think that they have merit in our age, or in any age, to some degree.) Nor is it that those values and ethics were always observed by those who were alive when such mores developed. My point is that the values and attitudes of the traditional martial Ways of Japan are different from the way we often tend to think and behave and that if we wish to understand and follow the budo, we must be aware of those differences, appreciate them, and put them in some perspective in our training and in our daily lives.

The budo were created as an integral part of Japanese culture. Saho, in turn, is an intrinsic aspect of the budo. To separate Japan's martial Ways from their parent culture is a waste of time, for the most part. To ignore the dimension of saho that runs so deeply through them is a thoughtlessly destructive error.

Part Two

CONTEMPLATING
TRADITION

12

TRADITION AND PERSONAL INTERPRETATION (*DENTO-KOSHO*)

"WE'RE 'TRADITIONALISTS,' so we don't change anything in the art."

For some, this kind of statement is considered a worthy, even noble sentiment. We picture the rugged conservator and preserver of ancient truths speaking this way, a person devoted to the continuation of an unbroken line of teachings in an art that has been forever enshrined, received in utterly perfect condition and in complete, unadulterated transmission. For others, such statements are the epitome of stuck-in-the mud intransigence. They are Ralph Waldo Emerson's "foolish consistency" that inevitably attends as a "hobgoblin of little minds."

"You 'traditionalists' are simply parroting something that may or may not have been an authentic formulation of an earlier era, aping techniques, preserving them as if they were museum pieces. And just as a stuffed auk or dodo will eventually become dusty and fragile, crumbling away into dry fragments, the 'specimen' of your technique will, over the generations, deteriorate and you will be left with nothing but an empty shell."

"No, no, you don't understand. We don't have the same perspective as the great masters of old. We don't have a good vantage point to see what was really going on in their training, and so we owe it to the art never to change a thing. If something in the art doesn't 'work,' it's because we haven't trained long or hard enough."

"Nonsense. You're dreaming. Waiting around for some divine 'secret' to appear that will give you special powers. You are using the step-by-step, 'don't deviate at all' approach to your training because you don't have the guts to look at the art critically and adapt it. You are killing it because you won't let it 'live.'"

Who's right? Hard to say. I tend to look at it the same way I look at LEGOs.

If you're a parent or a younger reader, you will be familiar with LEGOs. Lots of us are *very* familiar with them. Homes of young boys seem to be carpeted with the colorful little bricks. LEGOs are preformed plastic pieces that can be snapped together to make virtually anything. The number and varieties of LEGO pieces is astonishing. Staggering. There must be thousands of different kinds of them. What was even more surprising to me, when as a parent I began purchasing and assembling various LEGO kits, was the consistency in packaging. You can just buy LEGO pieces and build your own houses or towers or cars or whatever your imagination creates. The company, though, also sells kits that come with all the pieces—and just as crucially, the remarkably good instructions—to construct a LEGO world. From the Eiffel Tower to helicopters, race cars, and castles, there are LEGO kits to make scale reproductions. Some LEGO kits can contain up to four or five *thousand* pieces, all of which are designed to be assembled according to precise, multipage instruction booklets, into all those planes or pirate ships or dinosaurs or the Taj Mahal. You would assume, given the thousands of pieces and thousands of kits that must be assembled at the LEGO factory, that sooner or later, you'd buy one of these kits that is accidentally short a piece here or there. Having assembled several dozen of them when my child was a LEGO fanatic, I always tore open the packages with some trepidation, wondering what piece would have been left out, making the project come to a premature halt. It was amazing. I never once found a kit that was missing a single piece.

There are probably microcomputer chip manufacturers who don't have the quality control standards of a LEGO factory.

At any rate, I think LEGOs are a good metaphor for "traditionalism" in the martial arts. Like those kits, those arts that have withstood the test of time, generation after generation, are remarkably complete. (If all the parts of an art are not present, it isn't the fault of the art, usually, but rather the fault of the teacher who has not completely learned all aspects of that art before trying to teach it. This, as much as any other factor, is what's dysfunctional in the bulk of Japanese fighting arts today, in Japan and elsewhere in the world.) If you follow the "instruction book" of the typical Japanese martial art, you can build what that art intends to be built. That's not as simple as it sounds, however. First, if you've bought a LEGO kit that's meant to be assembled into the shape of a spaceship and you want to build a skyscraper, you're going to have some problems.

"I'm thinking about doing aikido because I'd like to be able to defend myself against multiple armed attackers," I heard a fellow say recently. Somehow, I doubt he'd generated this thought after talking with a competent aikido teacher. More likely he came up with it because of something he read or saw in a movie. In effect, he was thinking of picking up a LEGO kit, hoping to build a race car but not noticing on the box that this kit was for building a submarine. Perhaps there is an aikido teacher out there who professes to highlight this aspect of combat in his dojo and can deliver on that. I think, however, most aikido sensei would advise the fellow to look elsewhere. I have never seen an aikido dojo advertise this particular skill as the primary goal of their training. So someone entering an aikido dojo with that expectation is, like the person buying a LEGO submarine kit and hoping for a car, probably going to be disappointed. And that disappointment is hardly the fault of the aikido dojo, is it?

More to my point, though, again using the analogy of our LEGOs, is a feature of these toys that isn't always or immediately obvious. After you have spent time following the directions for the kits, assembling according to the instructions whatever model you've purchased, you will start to notice the ways the plastic blocks fit together. You can begin to see how many of what size are necessary for building other structures. Once, in essence, you know how the pieces fit together, you can begin to adapt them. You can assemble them into shapes other than those specifically explained in the instruction manual. Children skilled in LEGO construction can, almost spontaneously it seems, scrabble through a pile of LEGO pieces and come up with extraordinary creations. They can do this because they are so familiar with the basic ways LEGOs fit together that creative construction emerges without much thought as to basic techniques. They know how the pieces can be fit; they are free to use their imagination to create new forms. Do I really need to draw this analogy to a close? I think not. I think you get the point. I do need to add, however, one caveat to this analogy. While the potential for creating objects with LEGOs is tremendous and broad, it is not limitless. It is impossible to build, for example, a working barbecue pit with LEGOs, no matter how skilled the builder. The plastic's going to melt long before the ribs are grilled, right? Similarly, while Japanese combative traditions have a spectrum far wider and deeper than most imagine, they are not magic. They cannot be expanded infinitely. If you are looking for an art that will allow you to dodge bullets or become immortal, you are out of luck. If you are looking for an art that will make you fearless or that will solve all your personal problems, again, you are going to be disappointed. The budo cannot do any of that. They have limitations. Their capacities, nevertheless, are so remarkable that most of us following them will spend the rest of our lives in them before they are exhausted.

At any rate, *dento-kosho* is an expression in Japanese that applies here. *Dento* means "tradition." Interestingly, it is written with two characters: the first meaning "transmission," the second "heritage." In other words, "tradition," the tradition we're always talking about in some martial arts circles, exists only when it is passed down. A suit of armor behind glass in a museum isn't "tradition." It plays a part in tradition only when it is used, metaphorically or even literally, from one generation to the next. The same goes for martial arts. They aren't "traditional" if they are not transmitted. They are dead. Or at best, a stuffed taxidermy exhibit.

Kosho means "personal interpretation" or "insight." It is kosho that animates dento. It is our insight into the art, fortified correctly through years of training in the fundamentals, that allows dento to continue. Those following a traditional path then, are not doing it for the sake of tradition itself. Tradition is rather a means to an end. Tradition depends upon the continued contributions of personal insight into an art. Conversely, those personal insights and interpretation mean nothing if they are not grounded in the established traditions of the art. It is a cycle.

The notion that tradition and individual insight and personal interpretation are mutually exclusive is a curious one. Certainly that notion is not a part of any "traditional" Japanese art and never has been. Tradition and personal interpretation are, by necessity and by the very definition of an "art," martial or otherwise, absolutely vital in their harmony. If you don't believe me, spend some time with LEGOs.

13

REINVENTING THE WHEEL

I'M AN IDEA MAN, Chuck. Like, get this: I've been thinking . . . Take a bread bun. Slit it down the center. Stick a sausage inside. Decorate it with some kinda condiments, mustard or relish or whatever. You'd have a snack you could eat anywhere. Ballparks, picnics. I'll make a fortune. You don't think so? Well, I'm not even going to try to explain this other idea I have, one for an engine that runs on—don't tell anyone—*refined petroleum*.

In other arenas, this might pass for broad comedy. In the martial arts scene in this century, particularly in the West, it is an ironic fact of life. In most of Asia, the vast majority of those involved in combative disciplines find one that's available, one that suits them, and they do their best to learn it. (There are some incredible exceptions, however. Especially in Japan. You haven't really experienced the full range of human weirdness until you have seen some of the goofy martial arts "created" by wacky Japanese eccentrics.) Every now and then someone with special aptitude might gain some insights and make minor improvements in a fighting art. By minor, I hasten to add, I mean *minor*. For example, the benefits of weight training have been recognized by many budo teachers. In most cases they don't incorporate this into practice in the dojo, but they encourage their students to do it on their own. Some warm-up exercises that might have once been part of training, like duck-walking squats, have proved to cause injuries and so they have been dropped. With very few exceptions, these changes are not central or even important at all to the core curriculum of a budo.

This approach, of learning the budo as it has been passed down and instituting changes only in a peripheral way, seems to have worked well enough for many hundreds of years. That is not to suggest in any way that the budo are "perfect" and must never have any alterations. It is to suggest rather that changes occur only incrementally and only after practitioners have a thorough understanding of the arts. It is to suggest further that the core elements of a budo have evolved over a long period of time, have been tested, and should be considered very carefully before any alterations are even proposed. In the twenty-first century, though, a lot of us seem to prefer a different take on the whole subject. A great many people appear to believe that the accumulated knowledge of those established arts is dreadfully fragmentary; outdated at best. Many others seem to be completely unaware that such knowledge ever existed. It is this latter group that has unwittingly supplied so much amusement for us, and it is to them that we turn our attentions in this chapter.

The group of which I speak is entertaining for much the same reasons, I suppose, that we laugh at those cartoons where some poor dumb soul struggles and sweats madly to climb a daunting precipice, only to discover at the summit that someone else is sitting comfortably there already, having walked up a staircase on the other side of the mountain. There is humor in the displays of ignorant arrogance, a certain pathos in the stupidity of a fellow who expends enormous effort in trying to accomplish something that's already been done before and in most cases, better. Think if it, if you will, as a case of reinventing the wheel.

I read recently an article the subject of which its author (and unfortunately many of its readers as well, probably) clearly thought quite revolutionary and a tremendous breakthrough in martial arts concepts. He had discovered that, by an attention to proper timing, you could launch a counter, a kick or a punch or whatever, just as your opponent was beginning his own attack. Doing so was a nifty way to beat that opponent, the article noted. You don't even have to worry about a block. If your timing is right, you will hit him when he is vulnerable, concentrated so much on his own strike he won't even see yours coming. The author had even coined a term for this amazing discovery he'd made. It was something like "stop-time hitting," as I recall. (These types invariably concoct very keen names for their ideas. They mightn't recognize a wheel, but they'd know a rotational vehicular modem right away.)

"Stop-time hitting" is, I would be quick to admit, really a superb part of strategy. It is a valuable skill. We would owe a debt of gratitude to the fellow who was explaining it, except for one minor detail: it is something every traditional martial artist has known about for many generations. In Japanese, it is called *sen no sen,* a rough translation of which would be "early interval timing." A version of it is called *debana-waza,* an "advancing technique" that exploits the opponent's initiating motion. The point is, there are thousands of karateka, kendoka, and other martial artists already training in what this author "discovered." And most of them are probably better at it than is the guy who thinks he invented it.

Another fellow I read about was earnestly explaining his "redactive synchronicity theory." This consisted, if I was reading correctly, of simultaneously redirecting an opponent's attack and, with the same arm or foot, making your own attack in the same motion. He was happily convinced he had created a brilliant new combative innovation. Hardly. The concept of *kobo ichi*—"attack and defense are one"—or *oji-waza,* techniques blending defense with a simultaneous counter, are a common aspect of virtually every Japanese fighting art, modern or medieval. Even basic karate kata (which would doubtless be disdained by this farsighted chap as nonfunctional) contain numerous examples.

These "innovations" go on and on. Every *shodan* aikido student knows that a joint can be manipulated at more than one angle at the same time, making the lock more effective, and that the smaller the joint, the more immediate the pain response. But don't tell that to the various experts who think they have "discovered" this concept and who conduct seminars instructing in their allegedly newly minted ideas. The karateka does not practice long at all before being taught the difference between basic training stances and the more relaxed, upright postures used in free-sparring kumite. Yet obviously there are several would-be martial arts innovators out there who apparently did not stick around the dojo long enough before rushing off to make this remarkable "discovery" on their own.

Why do so many of these people work so hard at reinventing the wheel in the martial arts? It is partly because the accumulated knowledge of Asian combative arts is not comprehensively taught except in a minority of dojo. Let's face it; there just aren't that many good budo teachers out there. It's partly, too, because too many people interested in those arts are culturally arrogant, lazy, and insensitive. They are like the aspiring writer who begins by trying to create his own language. On one hand, it is admirable to display that kind of initiative and ambition. On the other, though, why would someone go to such lengths to acquire knowledge or insights that are already readily available?

The answer, of course, is that they are not actually that available. To learn these concepts the practitioner must submit himself to the rigors and discipline of the traditional dojo. He must be patient and perceptive and persevering. This is, I'm afraid, not at all to the liking of the kinds of individuals we have been discussing. So they go off on their own. And that's what is most amusing, if you think about it. Because in trying to avoid effort, in looking for shortcuts on the path to combative effectiveness, they actually wind up working harder than they would have had to if they had just stuck it out in the dojo.

Maybe you don't find it all that amusing. Maybe you don't look forward with a smile for that revelation from the next self-taught master that, hey, guess what? The open hand is more versatile for striking than the fist, or that, gee, look at this: throwing techniques are more effective if you rotate your hips. Oh well. Maybe then, you'd be interested in a little innovation I've been thinking about. I call it the "digital video disc" ...

14

TAKABAKARI AND TAKING MEASUREMENT THE OLD FASHIONED WAY

IF YOU CONSIDER Japan's very long period of civil war, which lasted from the fourteenth through the seventeenth centuries, it is understandable that a great many weapons would have developed. Warriors were always looking for the extra edge an unusual or unique weapon might give them. An opponent who had never encountered that weapon before would be at a distinct disadvantage in a fight. In the period following Japan's civil war, combative arts found practical application in duels or matches between practitioners or schools, and again, not surprisingly, this led to an even more varied development of weaponry. It was this period that led to the creation of the *kusarigama* (sickle and weighted chain), the *jutte* (a forked truncheon), and other sorts of "oddball" weapons that would have been of little use on a battlefield but that were excellent for dueling or self-defense or law enforcement.

The use of many of these weapons has survived, though rarely in practical form as a method of self-defense or for employment on the battlefield. Rather, these weapons are preserved and studied today as a kind of "living artifact," a physical way of looking into the past and discovering how the warrior class of old Japan fought, how they thought about combat, and how they approached it from a technological point of view.

In probably the majority of *ryu,* or classical traditions, that continue to teach these weapons, the dimensions of the weapon itself are fixed and standardized. If I am a member of the Shibukawa ryu and learning their jutte techniques, the jutte I and every other member will use will be identical. Same dimensions, weight—even the exact place the forked tine is molded to the shaft is standard for that ryu. The same is true for the *bo,* the long staff used in the Tatsumi ryu. The ryu's teachings call for a specific length of the weapon. This leads to a worthwhile inquiry, especially when we consider arts like these as practiced today: What if my hands are much larger than the original practitioners using that jutte? What if I am shorter or taller than the Tatsumi ryu masters of old? Why can't I modify the length of my weapons accordingly? Indeed, why would I *not* want to do this, modify and personalize the weapon to suit my size better?

In some cases there are reasons particular to a ryu why this cannot happen. They may have strategies or techniques in which the dimensions of a weapon, especially its length, are critical. In others, some principles are best taught with a certain size weapon, and while the practitioner might have been free, once having internalized those principles, to select a different size, during his training he was expected to use the standard model. In other ryu, however, the answer to the question of "why can't I individualize my weapon?" is "why of course you can." In many ryu and with many weapons, individualization was common. And in many cases, the way it was determined is interesting. It was done through what's called *takabakari.* Takabakari is the old Japanese custom of measuring things according to dimensions of the human body. The unit of measure called a *sun,* for instance, was defined, roughly, by the distance between your fingertip and its first joint. (Karateka will be familiar with this word; it's used in *sun-dome,* the stopping—*dome*—of an attack, for safety in training's sake, one *sun* from the target.) A *shaku* was the length between the wrist and elbow. (Readers with experience in a Japanese or Okinawan staff art will recognize this measure in *rokushaku-bo,* a staff of six shaku.) Each practitioner customized the dimensions, especially the length, of his weapons according to the measurements of his own body.

Stick weapons were often measured by takabakari. A *mimikiri-bo* was determined by the height of the user's ear, a *chigiri-bo* by the height of his breast, a *koshikiri-bo* by the height of his hip. (We find this form of individualized measurement, incidentally, in certain Chinese staffs as well, as with the "eyebrow stick.") In each of these terms is the character for "cut," or *kiri*. So the ear-length bo was cut at the height of the user's *mimi*, or ear, and so on. The *hijikiri-bo* was a weapon cut to measure from the elbow (*hiji*) of the user to a point somewhere along his hand. In some ryu like the Toda ryu, the length was measured from the elbow to the tip of the extended middle finger; in others, it might be to the base of the wrist. Today, one often hears of *tanbo* (short stick) or *hanbo* (half stick) in Japanese weapon arts. There is no "official" measurement for these sticks. What exactly constituted a "half stick" would depend entirely on the length of what a full-size *bo* (sometimes referred to as a *cho-bo,* or "long bo") was called for in a particular ryu. Often, however, both these weapons will be sized individually through takabakari: the tanbo being some variation of the elbow-to-hand ratio; the hanbo, an approximation of the measurement between the ground and a user's hip or navel.

It doesn't relate directly to the topic of takabakari, but a common question when the subject is feudal Japanese weaponry, by the way, is about the distinction between a bo and a *jo*. Most students know a jo is shorter than a bo, but when does the former become long enough to be classified as the latter? There is no definitive answer. Some schools using a stick would call it a bo, while others, using one roughly the same length, would refer to it as a jo. As a very general rule, some practitioners in the old days and today consider a jo a stick short enough to be manipulated to strike with one end and then the other in a single motion. A bo is long enough there must be an intermediary movement when going from the proximal to the distal end.

Returning to takabakari: *tegiribo* were among the shortest weapons in the arsenal of old Japan: sticks that are, as the name implies "cut" to the length of the *te,* or hand. (This is a good example of what we just noted above. The stick here is less than a foot long, yet in most classical schools that used it, it was called a bo.) They could be the length of the distance between the outstretched tip of the little finger and the thumb or be as long as the bottom of the wrist to the tip of the middle finger. They were held in the closed fist for striking at *kyusho* or vital points, or they could be fitted between the fingers to make joint locks more effective and painful.

Aside from its value as a curiosity from another age, the matter of takabakari is of little practical interest to today's martial artist, to be sure. But two points regarding it are worthwhile for consideration. First, the individualized methods for determining an effective length of a weapon during an age when they were actually used in combat highlights the emphasis the classical warrior placed on practicality. Contrary to popular assumptions about the rigidity of his arts, the fighting man was not blindly loyal to a standardized way of looking at his equipment or his arts. He recognized the need to be flexible and to modify things if necessary. Second, we should consider a similar approach to our own training. An uncritical reliance on dogma or inflexible standards is perhaps useful for a certain stage of learning. Rote learning, just trying to absorb the lessons uncritically and doing it "because Sensei says so," is sufficient until we gain a deeper understanding of a practice. As one advances in a realistic combative art, however, this attitude can become robotic and stale. Always under the guidance of a qualified teacher, we eventually have to begin to make the art our own.

15

SECRETS

THERE ARE—I read this stuff on Internet sites and get letters from readers who bring it up frequently—two kinds of "secrets," or shall we say, "privileged information," in martial arts schools. And we need to be very clear about the differences between them.

Suzuki Sensei and his senior student Smith have been teacher and student for years. Smith has, with Suzuki's blessings, gone off to start his own dojo in another city. Suddenly, Suzuki calls together all his other senior students and announces, "Smith is no longer in our organization. No one will be allowed to train with him. His rank and status are revoked." And that's the end of it. Perhaps Smith has cheated Suzuki financially. Maybe he's behaved immorally. Everyone wonders. I, a complete outsider, ask on an online budo forum, "What gives?" I will be politely told the matter of Smith and Suzuki is none of my business. And it isn't, no more than the reason a couple who have lived two streets over in my neighborhood suddenly get a divorce. It's a private matter. Let's say, however, that one of that couple is my cousin or my nephew. In that case, it is a family matter. And I would not be out of place to start calling other family members to ask, "What happened with Will and Mary?"

The same is true for senior students of Suzuki. Suzuki owes me, a stranger, nothing. He does, however, owe his students an explanation, just as my nephew or cousin would, directly or communicated through other family members, owe me an explanation about a sudden divorce. The idea that a close relative could simply announce one day over the holiday table that he's divorced and we are all supposed to just nod and go back to our meal is preposterous. Similarly, it is absurd for Suzuki to just announce the expulsion of a longtime student, a senior in his organization, without explanation to the other seniors. (We're not talking about sharing the explanation with the whole group necessarily. We are talking, remember, about seniors who have some standing in the organization.) And don't try to tell me that's the "traditional Japanese way." I am a senior member of two different classical martial ryu, both more than four centuries old. And if either of my teachers kicked someone out of the ryu, I would immediately go to other seniors to find out why, and if they didn't know, any or all of us would go to our teacher and ask him directly. And he would tell us. It's that simple. And I would never consider training under the sort of leadership who didn't give me that consideration. I would also suspect his refusal to talk about it implied serious questions about his integrity, no matter how skilled a technical teacher he is.

That's one kind of secret, a secret in the sense that outsiders might not be privy to the details and would have no legitimate reason to be, but one that would be shared and kept in confidence by senior members of the ryu or organization. Here's another kind of secret, though, one I'm hearing about and which is being confused with the sort of privileged information we have just discussed.

Let's say Suzuki Sensei's teacher was a guy named Oyama, or so Suzuki has claimed in articles or books or public presentations. Trouble is, there is no historical evidence that Oyama ever existed. True, there are all kinds of stories about him, about where he lived and when. But there is no independent verification that he was a real person. In this case, if I chime in with questions about Oyama on a forum or in some publication, it is *not* appropriate to be told that's none of my business. In this case, a historical fact has been presented publicly. Historians, researchers, all kinds of martial arts enthusiasts have a legitimate interest in that fact, whether they are members of Suzuki's organization or not. Let's say Suzuki claims to have trained in some ryu no one's ever heard of. Again, it is not a reasonable answer, when the history or particulars of this ryu are questioned, to be told "That's none of your business." If such information is kept entirely within the group and considered privileged, fine. But don't present it publicly and then behave as if it is intrusive when questions about it are raised.

To be sure, especially with classical martial arts dating back centuries, some figure claimed as a member or headmaster might be tough to prove as a historical reality. And there are matters not discussed with nonmembers. The ryu or group will admit all that to anyone who inquires. I cannot think of a single martial art or ryu, however, that would consider historical records or lineages to be proprietary information within the ryu. They never have been. Quite the opposite. I have visited the dojo of martial ryu in Japan where the teacher or headmaster will happily drag out boxes of scrolls and unroll them for inspection. These individuals regularly cooperate with historians and writers. The *techniques* of a school might well be secret. The history of that school? Nope.

When Suzuki is not honest about his past or his lineage or the history of the art or school he is teaching, there is inevitably a depressing consequence among his followers. They are forced into the pathetic role of apologists. Often we see them trying valiantly to defend, to equivocate, to make wild guesses or outlandish theories that attempt to explain away the discrepancies. Criticism, fair and unfair, along with sincere inquiries, are all lumped together in their minds as attacks. Frequently, lacking facts, they will lash out with vicious ad hominem arguments. Finally, either at Suzuki's orders or on their own, they simply close ranks and retire from any further discussion. This is often painted among themselves as a noble retreat. "We know the truth. We know what a wonderful guy Suzuki is. We're too busy training to participate in silly discussions." This is sad. And it is dangerous, in that it replaces reason and a respect for independent truth for a kind of semireligious, almost cultish in some cases, belief system.

In many significant ways, budo is about a confrontation with truth. Every time we step into the dojo it is an opportunity to strip away illusions—especially the self-crafted kind—to see reality. Incessantly we have to deal with the temptation to do otherwise. "I'd have passed my *shodan* test but Sensei doesn't like me." "I trained extra hard last week so I can skip class tonight." "I look out of shape, but I'm really developing my inner ki power." Excuses. Equivocation. Self-induced illusions. Until we can recognize these for what they are and for the limits they necessarily impose on us, we cannot get very far along any serious martial path. When you are met with lies or obfuscation about a central aspect of your art—the reality of its history—it is hardly a promising sign you will go very far in confronting other realities.

There are those who insist any concern with the past, whether it be in the lineage or history of a combative art, is at best a distraction. Why care who my teacher's teacher was? I can see, from a pragmatic point of view, that what I'm learning is effective and worthwhile to me and enjoyable. So if Sensei doesn't want to talk about some stuff, who cares? It is a reasonable argument. I don't need to know from what waters it swam in or the name of the guy who caught it to know the cod I'm eating tonight is good, nutritious, and safe for consumption. Knowing the name of some art my teacher may have studied half a century ago isn't going to protect me from the Glock that mugger's about to stick in my face. That's all true. It is also true that knowing Babe Ruth's batting average or the history of the strike zone isn't going to make you a better ball player. Nevertheless, there are historians and researchers who are interested in that and denying the legitimacy of their interest or stonewalling their inquiries is ridiculous.

Demanding to know some intimate detail of the private life of your favorite pitcher is not the same as asking about the history of his team. Asking the first question is intrusive and rude. Refusing to answer the second is weird and troubling.

16

HOW COME THEY FOUGHT
DIFFERENTLY IN THE OLD DAYS?

"THAT TRADITIONAL STUFF doesn't work in a real street fight situation." How many times, and in how many variations, have you heard this? It is offered as advice or an opinion, on a drearily predictable schedule now. We hear it constantly, as we also hear those now who speak authoritatively about "reality based" methods of combat. (As opposed, one must assume, to those disciplines devoted to "unreality.") Interestingly, I never hear or read anyone wonder just why it is that traditional stuff doesn't work, and if ever it did, when, exactly, it became obsolete. Apparently, many critics of "traditional stuff" believe there was a time in the hazy past when bad guys cocked a fist against their side, then cut loose with a straight punch that could be effectively blocked by a defender in his perfect front stance. Somehow, these critics must believe, "street fight situations" at one time looked like a basic karate class. When was this? When did thugs and muggers and brawlers make straightforward punches or those convenient lapel grabs that allowed for neat jujutsu tricks to be used as counters?

If we follow the logic of these critics, we must suppose that around the mid-1970s, when "full contact" fighting came into vogue, someone woke up one morning and realized "real" fighting involved a lot of grappling and head butts and gouging and multiple, simultaneous attacks. Wow. How brilliant these innovators must have been to have found this truth and to have set about to rectify matters.

It is typical of some people, mostly those of an adolescent mentality, to believe that nothing important has happened unless it has been in their lifetimes. They seem to believe that until the advent of grappling, contact-type combative sports, fighting arts consisted of delusional dweebs attired in pajamas throwing jerky, unrealistic kicks and punches, and, of course, "judo chops" at one another. And we would have to conclude that all those "traditionalists" were either involved in a massive, cultlike self-deception or that bad guys back then were just really, really stupid and easily defeated by such methods.

The truth is, people engaged in hand-to-hand fighting, whether on a battlefield or in a bar, tend to go at it in much the same way they always have. Physiologically, we have not changed in several thousand years. True, culture plays a role in how we fight. I remember when anyone who kicked in a fight would be labeled a "sissy." Criminals and bullies as well as cops and ordinary citizens are very apt to include kicking in their attacks and defenses now. And expectations about fighting play a role as well. An English schoolboy engaged in fisticuffs a century ago could expect that his opponent would accept defeat if his nose was bloodied. City gangs back in the 1950s often had elaborate rituals of approaching one another, almost stalking, and doing lots of posturing. Now that gang violence often starts with a car driving by and spraying gunfire, those rituals have disappeared. Gang members are criminals, but they aren't stupid for the most part. They adapted their behavior to meet a change in combat. Some Southeast Asian forms of combat have ceremonial aspects about them that are almost as important as the fighting, and so this influences their methods, especially when the fight is between individuals who share the same culture. Practical aspects of daily life can also influence personal combat. Feudal Japanese arts, for instance, didn't include a lot of kicking, simply because kimonos and *hakama* make kicking more difficult.

Those, however, are secondary considerations in most ways.

When it comes down to individuals engaged in personal combat, hand to hand, we haven't suddenly discovered anything new. That's why it is silly to talk about "traditional" methods of fighting. Rather than compare so-called traditional and "reality" combat disciplines, it is more appropriate to think of a distinction in *approaches* to learning to fight. Certainly it is true there are superior and inferior ways of teaching and learning fighting. The karate dojo where kata is perceived as a rote exercise, performed robotically and always against an imaginary opponent, is not engaging in traditional training. It is more accurately engaging in inferior training, probably led by someone who never learned correctly in the first place and who is now passing down bad habits and training methods to his students. The grappling school where students go to the mat immediately and are instructed in a haphazard way that never introduces or practices fundamentals, always hoping to "find out what works" in the heat of the action, is not really doing anything new and revolutionary. It is just bad training, not unlike tossing someone off a pier to teach them to learn to swim. There really isn't much different between these two schools, even though both may think of themselves as opposite ends of the spectrum.

What passes for traditional fighting arts training, especially in the arena of the Japanese combative arts, is a stylized pantomime in far too many schools. But just because I am doing some diluted form of something I'm calling karate or judo, and consequently it is a miserable failure when tested in real life, does not mean karate or judo are unrealistic. It was my approach to these arts that was not realistic. To believe otherwise is to embrace the weird logic that karate, from its earliest evolution in seventeenth-century Okinawa right up until the present, has been an enormous fraud. That judo is little more than a century and a half's exercise in self-delusion. It "worked" in the past. If it doesn't now, it isn't because people have learned to fight differently. It is more likely because you aren't doing it right.

The objection to my logic here would be that I am blaming the victim: It might seem that I continue to hold karate or judo or any budo as some kind of magically powerful art, and if it fails to work, why, it cannot be the fault of my beloved martial Ways. No, it must be you who have failed. The flaw in that criticism is that neither I nor any other responsible practitioner or exponent of any martial Way has ever held them to be magic or indomitable. Fighting is a dangerous, unpredictable enterprise. If karate or any other fighting art was a foolproof way of always winning, always avoiding injury, it would be practiced universally and with complete enthusiasm by anyone who might ever have to resort to violence. It isn't. Karate is one approach, one way of confronting confrontation and physical danger in the form of combat. It isn't without limitations, and there are even more limitations placed on its effectiveness by the dedication, understanding, and innate talent of those who practice it. Much the same can be said for any other method or style of fighting.

One chooses to follow a martial Way not because it is perfect or incomparable or flawlessly reliable. One follows a budo because it is a serious way of engaging and confronting violence, a way that has obviously been proven over the many, many years in which it has been practiced. One follows a particular budo rather than some other kind of fighting art because that budo has particular and specific attractions, ethical and cultural and aesthetic, that appeal to some. If those attractions begin to outweigh its practical combative applications in the training of some of its followers, that can have consequences, good and bad.

You can believe, of course, that they just didn't know how to fight in the old days as well as we do now. You can believe "traditional martial arts" are somehow outmoded and that their masters and practitioners in the past never had to deal with the threats or techniques we have today. You can, if you wish, be pleased that it is your generation that's discovered truths about personal combat that the old-timers never realized. And that you have witnessed or participated in a new and unique creation in the long history of conflict. Congratulations.

17

THE IMPORTANCE OF A GOOD TEACHER

TEACHER IS A THREE-HOUR drive from your home, meaning you can only go to train with him two or three times a month? Okay. You'll learn more slowly. And there will be frustrating visits to his dojo when you do not learn any new material but instead must be corrected on what you have already learned—or more accurately, *mislearned.*

Teacher old? You will tend to start moving the way he does. Your movements will become smaller, shorter, in places where they should be big and long. That's troublesome. I have seen dojo where twenty-something guys—young, agile, strong men—move around like they are only months away from a walker. Unconsciously or deliberately, they copy the posture and movements of the older teacher, even if he tells them not to. However, in a good dojo, you can overcome that. There will be younger, more active seniors who will step in and correct you, and your teacher himself will start criticizing you. "Are you as old as me? Why are you moving like you are?!"

School or work preventing you from training as often as you would like? That's tough, but you must remember that family, education, and work should all come before your budo training. Again, you may not learn as fast as you would like. But again, too, with patience, you will get there and the teacher will be there to lead you.

In short, training under a good teacher isn't always a perfect situation. There are often obstacles that will be encountered. Some are tough to overcome. Most, however, can be, with the right spirit and the necessary patience. Overcoming a poor teacher, though, is something else.

Plainly put, you have virtually no chance in budo of overcoming the obstacles and limitations of a poor teacher.

Nearly all the problems we have with martial arts today (and there *are* a lot of them) can be traced back to poor teaching. I do not necessarily mean teachers who are inadequate because they pretend to have skills they don't or who teach because it satisfies some weird ego problem they have—although, of course, there are plenty of those. There are also teachers, however, who are honest, well-meaning, utterly dedicated—but they are, nonetheless, still poor teachers.

Let me posit two concepts that explain this. First, it is immensely, extremely difficult to teach a budo. Second, there are very, *very* few people who are really qualified to do it.

We are apt to take it for granted that budo is really fairly easy to teach and learn so long as one has the physical and mental stamina to stick with it. After all, there are dojo by the thousands, all over the country. And there are thousands of teachers, in dojo, community centers, and so on, who are leading classes. The truth, however, is that the Japanese martial Ways are enormously, dauntingly sophisticated. They are ferociously hard to learn, harder still to teach. Most people don't get that.

I learned the mechanics of the wrist throw last month. Had it explained, practiced it. Now I can teach it. This sounds like a reasonable conclusion. But in fact, being able to produce a wrist throw and understanding its mechanics *as they relate to you* does not mean you can reproduce it in someone else. That person has a different body. They may encounter different problems learning a wrist throw you didn't have. Possessing the understanding of the wrist throw on a level where you can deal with these situations takes years of training and experience and insight. In the same sense, learning a wrist throw while working in a comfortable environment with a cooperative practice partner is one thing. Learning the timing to employ the throw, the methods to set it up effectively, the coordination to use the wrist throw in combination with other movements: these are extraordinarily difficult lessons. The reality is that most of the budoka who learn skills like the wrist throw easily and well have a natural talent to be able to teach themselves. They learn not *because* of a teacher but *in spite* of that teacher.

The teacher needs to do much more than just learn how to perform a wrist throw before he can teach it. He needs to understand the underlying principles of his particular form of budo. He needs to grasp the principles of his art so thoroughly that he can see how they are embodied in any of its techniques. And he must be able to understand the reverse. He must know how the particular—the wrist throw in this case—reflects the general principles of his art, how the throw is consistent with and reinforces those vital principles. In this way, he can begin to teach the foundations of the art as a whole instead of just instructing in disparate, unconnected techniques. While it seems obvious, an inability to understand the general principles of an art is a widespread problem in the budo. It is why so many "teachers" actually just instruct a mishmash of disparate techniques and strategies, hoping to cobble them together in a "best of" collection of different arts they have learned. These teachers fail to understand that viable fighting arts must be based on coherent principles that organize the body and the mind in a way that is dependable and capable of being integrated as a whole into the individual. Imagine, in a crisis, a shooter who has been trained by one instructor how to use the front sights of his gun to aim and been taught by another teacher to shoot instinctively. He's going to be confused, disorganized. The budoka who doesn't have a consistency in his art is no different.

Interpreting the martial Ways as a tool bag of basically unrelated techniques, teaching them without any sense of connection, unfortunately is common. The reality is that any budo demands a certain perspective in order to be communicated effectively. The person who would be a teacher has to climb to a point where his view is sufficiently broad in order to show others how to get to where he is and to go beyond. Even with such a teacher, it isn't easy. Without one? Good luck.

18

TEACHERS AND STUDENTS

HOW MANY STUDENTS does a teacher have? How many—if by "teacher" we are talking about a budo sensei—*can* he have? Is there a limit to the number of students one person can legitimately and competently instruct?

Some training halls boast of several scores of students. Some have even more. A friend brings to my attention the yearly gross of a local martial arts instructor: nearly half a million dollars. He has to do the math for me, but it comes out that the number of students this instructor would have needed would have been in the thousands, a concept quite staggering to me. Given that the instructor teaches in a facility that was once a large K-Mart-type store and drives a Mercedes that matches another driven by his wife, I'm told, I don't doubt the income level. Some of these places even use the vast number of their students and members as a part of their advertising. I guess that works. I'm not sure I would be all that excited about signing on to become a client of a doctor or a lawyer who advertised that people were waiting in lines around the block to get in, since I don't think I would exactly be getting up-close and personal service. But I am willing to acknowledge people might be motivated to go to those martial arts megaschools for different reasons than those compelling them to seek a lawyer or physician.

An aikido teacher I know once said with some honesty that not all those who trained with him were his students. That's interesting, isn't it? I think perhaps what the teacher meant was that just paying one's training fees and attending classes does not mean the student is entitled to be guaranteed a place in the teacher's serious consideration. Apparently, the teacher meant that the dojo member had to earn his attention and particular interest. This, after all, the aikido teacher went on to explain, is how things were done in the "old days." That's true, sort of. In many—though not all by any means—feudal-era schools, there weren't many students, and the inner teachings of a ryu might be passed on to only a very few. But the sensei in these ryu didn't take money for instruction and then deny that those he was instructing were his students, either. (Note: Warning bells go off for me whenever I hear a teacher of modern budo talk about the old days. Even if they are Japanese, coming directly from the native culture of the budo, I am wary. Often, they tend to rely on childhood memories of TV's afternoon samurai drama more than anything else for their information. Only a small minority of Japanese budo sensei have even seen classical martial arts; fewer still have had any training in them that would give them a realistic glimpse of what the "old days" of budo were actually like. For the most part, their version of these old days, in addition to romantic fiction, is a rehash of pre–World War II militarism with a bit of collegiate budo-club sadism and bullying thrown in.)

It is certainly possible to see the aikido teacher's perspective on this. If I were a budo teacher, I might take the same position. Pay your fees and you have access to the dojo and to some kind of instruction, whether from me or from one of my seniors. Stay long enough and show enough initiative and drive and eventually I'll begin to notice you, and stay long enough after that and I will begin to consider you my student. Fair enough. But if I were to take that path in instructing, I hope I would be honest enough to tell prospective and beginner students all about my perspective up front.

Even if we accept that not all those training under the direction of a sensei—I resist the urge to call them "customers" here, but just barely—are not specifically his students, the question remains of just how many a teacher can truly have. The question is instructive. So, too, is how each of us would answer it. I once met the senior student of a well-known karate teacher here in the United States. This fellow had trained with his sensei for twenty years. Of the literally thousands of students who had come and gone, this student was among the very few who had stuck it out. He started his training with his teacher when the teacher just arrived from Japan. Making conversation, I asked what kind of home the sensei lived in. I don't know, the student said. I've never been there. He was surprised at my surprise. How could you spend two decades in a relationship as close as the one between teacher and student, longer than most marriages in this country, and never even have been in the guy's house? The fellow had met his teacher's wife once, seen the teacher's children a few times. That was pretty much the scope of his interaction with the sensei's life outside the dojo. Perhaps I am naive, but I wonder how much I, if I were a teacher, could influence you if in twenty years together our relationship was one where the occasion to get to know my spouse and child had never arisen.

Was this fellow a student of the sensei? Indisputably, in some ways. But it is hard for me to fathom how, in others. In some ways, every person who comes in contact with a teacher, I suppose, if that person is seeking instruction, can be said to have been a student of that teacher. Sometimes the teacher will do or say something, just a momentary exchange quite forgotten by the teacher five minutes later, that will have a profound, fundamental effect on the student for years to come. It's possible. It is possible, too, to have been teaching a student for twenty years and never have any significant influence on him at all. Interesting perspectives and points to consider on the whole matter, which, I daresay, should concern both teachers and students and which should have some resonance in a wide range of matters. What is your motivation in seeking a teacher? What is your motivation in teaching?

And in the end, the answer to my initial question may be that the teacher might never know how many students he has had. Or how few.

19

SOUL BUDO

WHEN I WAS A KID and was around a lot of older college guys from Hawaii, the subject of surfing often came up. Many of my seniors in budo were surfers. This was back in the sixties, when surfing was still an amateur diversion. Hawaii had a few local competitions. But the days of pro surfing, with corporate sponsors and full-time surfers, was still way off in the future. Even then, though, I remember hearing about guys who called themselves "soul surfers." They used the term to distinguish themselves from the surfers who entered competitions to have their rides judged by a panel and who collected trophies and championships. Soul surfers liked to define themselves by their purity and their ideals. They surfed, they insisted, for the art of it all.

I thought of those soul surfers recently when an old friend wrote to tell me of his experience of getting back into karate after having left it for more than twenty years. He is nearly sixty now, and he would be the first to admit that a lot of couch-camping has diminished his stamina and strength. Still, he's determined to go as far as he can. He wants to retrace the steps along the Way he took earlier in life and, if possible, perhaps even to go past where he was before. Age and its limitations can slow one's steps on this path. But the added wisdom and insights of maturity can make the journey more rewarding as well.

"I can judge my own progress and I don't care about testing," he told me.

I would agree with him wholeheartedly on the whole testing mess that has come to be a feature of karate and all the other budo. The more rank tests have become institutionalized as a part of budo training, the more vulnerable these arts have become to rot and to the insincerity of overcommercialism. Do you really think there is a noticeable, objective difference between a third-kyu and a first-kyu, for example? Testing has encouraged teachers to become stingy. If I give my student a rank that allows him to test people himself, those people no longer come to me to pay their testing fees. They go to my authorized student, depriving me of the income they represent. Naturally, placing all this emphasis on testing also cheats students by encouraging them to look at promotions as a real measure of their progress.

I would disagree, however, when my friend says he can judge his own progress. I doubt it. I have written probably more than anyone about the hypocrisy of modern budo ranking systems and their abuse. However, criticizing the unsavory elements attending to the ranking process is not the same as criticizing the system itself.

The surfers out there waiting to catch a wave, disdaining competitions, in it only for the love of it all, can argue a precedent of sorts. The native Hawaiians who originated the sport didn't leave any record of contests. So the soul surfer might have a point in saying he's returning to a purer moment in wave riding. The karateka who makes the same claim about karate training, however—that he wants to go back to a golden era when one trained simply for the spiritual love of the art—is, in historical terms, easily dumped into the ocean.

If you are recalling the age of Okinawan karate, before it was transplanted to the Japanese mainland, then of course, there were no *kyu-dan* ranking systems. Nobody wore black belts or green or purple ones. If you are training under one of those rare systems that has resisted or eschewed a ranking system, one of Okinawan origin, then you won't ever deal with rank. The fact is, however, that all Japanese karate systems and the vast majority of Okinawan schools have adopted ranks. They did so going back to the early part of the twentieth century. There is some "traditional" karate that may not include ranks or testing. But these are rare systems. Unless you are a member of one of them, you will be faced with ranks and with testing for them. The same can be said of all the other forms of modern budo. Judo, aikido, kendo, *kyudo, naginata-do*: it is impossible to name a budo form that has not always included some kind of ranking in its curriculum.

Sure, if you are getting something from your training, that's good. It might be improved fitness. It might be that you enjoy the camaraderie of the dojo. You feel better about yourself by being a part of the group. The budo may also be beneficial for you in terms of adding a spiritual element to your life. You may sense that your ability to handle stressful situations, including those that may involve violence, is enhanced by following a martial Way. But here's the point: if you undertake budo practice, you don't get to choose what part of it you will do and what part you won't. It isn't like a cafeteria. You don't get to pick and choose. "I'll spar, but I won't do kata." "I will train with other women but men frighten me so I'd prefer not to have them as practice partners."

That is the sort of attitude that spells almost certain failure in budo. It is the attitude that, if allowed in a dojo, almost certainly sets the stage for the failure of the dojo. You cannot have students deciding what aspects of their training they will participate in and those they will take a pass on. Budo organizations have ranking protocol for a reason. As a beginner, you may not understand the reason. With more experience, you may understand it and still not like or agree with it. Doesn't matter. If you want to be part of that school, that organization, that system, then you accept it as it is. You may, if you advance far enough, eventually be in a position to modify some aspects of the school. You may even be able to advance to a point of authority where you can eliminate testing or ranks altogether.

Right now, though, you owe it to the school and the system and your teacher to do as he asks.

There are some ways in which you may judge your own progress in the dojo. There are others in which you must, if you are serious about your training, rely on those above you. Trust them. If you do not, don't train with them. Don't think you understand the "soul" of budo and can therefore decide what's good and bad about your art. If you really want to see its soul, immerse yourself with a good school and teacher. It is the only way to make real progress.

20

LICENSED TO KILL—OR SOMETHING

THE SERIOUS BUDOKA should understand something about the ranking system in modern budo and how it came to be—and where it might be going.

As most practitioners know, the *dan-i* or *dan* ranking system is relatively recent in all Japanese martial arts. Near the turn of the last century, judo's founder, Jigoro Kano, gave black belts to some of his senior students, distinguishing them from lesser-experienced judoka, who wore white belts. In the early twentiety century, Mikonosuke Kawaishi, who introduced judo to France, devised the series of colored belts familiar today. He also instituted the practice of having students learn part of a certain, set curriculum, then testing them on it and awarding a particular belt for their efforts. The belt signifies a "promotion" in the art. This method of grading was quickly adopted by karate-do in Japan and, later, by aikido. Some modern martial arts like kendo and iaido adopted the dan-i method of grading, issuing certificates but not colored belts. Other Japanese arts, like some schools of calligraphy and the board game of *go,* also employed the dan-i system. Grades in this system are kyu and dan. Kyu ranks are for relative beginners and run from a specific highest number up to the lowest. So a fourth kyu has a lower grading than a first kyu. Dan ranks, for more senior practitioners (and marked in most budo by the black belt), conversely, go up. A fifth dan, for example, is higher ranked than a second dan.

Prior to the dan-i awarding of rank, classical Japanese arts relied primarily on the *den-i* system, which is not really a grading per se but is rather best thought of as a kind of licensing. The den-i is a product of the ryu. The ryu is, for lack of a better analogy, something like a pyramid scheme. The headmaster is at the top. It is he or one of his ancestors who has identified a specific principle, a coherent, distinctive body of technique. He teaches this and has the exclusive right to control it, and when he feels students have acquired sufficient skill and understanding of the particular elements of the art, he recognizes this by giving them *menkyo,* or "licenses." Sometimes the license allows the student to teach all or part of the art. In that case, the student becomes a teacher as well, instructing yet continuing to rely on his teacher and to recognize him as the top of the structure. This is the fundamental nature of all ryu, whether they are devoted to martial arts or to Noh theater or tea ceremony or flower arranging.

While many modern karate organizations use *ryu* in their title, virtually none of them meet the classical definition of the word. In fact, no modern budo can really be thought of as a traditional ryu. Most modern budo organizations are more like sports federations, run more like corporations, with boards and committees and so on. This is a natural evolution and a necessary one given the size of the average martial arts organization, with members worldwide and hundreds of instructors. It does lead to problems, however, as when the founder of the organization, usually Japanese, will veer from trying to act like the CEO of a modern corporation to behaving like the feudal headmaster of a ryu, all within the space of a single meeting. Budo organizations are still in the painful process of sorting out and coming to terms with the modern age, reconciling these realities with a feudal past.

The member of a feudal ryu did not, of course, receive a colored belt, or a "promotion," in the sense that today's karateka or judoka does. Ryu were mostly small, regionally centralized groups. As a member, you probably lived within walking distance of your teacher's home and were related, through family or clan ties, to most of the other ryu members. In this setting, your relationship with your teacher was much closer than in the average dojo of today. Evaluating your progress and your skill did not require a test. The teacher had a good idea of where you were and what you knew. At some point, he would elect to recognize this, presenting you with a license.

Each ryu had its own system of licensing. Among the most common were *kirigami,* a paper, sometimes cut or folded in a distinctive way, upon which was written the license. *Makimono,* or scrolls, were also used. In some cases, these documents contained a list, or *mokuroku,* of the techniques of the school. They might also detail what or how much of the curriculum the recipient was permitted to teach. The headmaster of a ryu might also possess scrolls that were not technically licenses but, rather, contained the secret principles of the art. These were usually written in flowery, poetic language that would have had little meaning unless one had been initiated into the teachings of the school. They would be passed on to the next generation of headmaster. In some ryu, a *menkyo-kaiden* or similar license might be issued that would grant the recipient full authority to teach and represent the ryu. Today, those classical ryu still in existence use the den-i as a way of recognizing authority and teaching within the ryu.

The modern dan-i and the classical den-i have something in common in that they are valid gradings or licensing within the structure of the ryu or the organization. That's important. If I am a *sandan,* a third dan in the Mushi-kera style of karate, that rank, of course, will mean nothing to another karate organization. They will have different grading standards. Further, let us say I do something thought reprehensible: I steal from the dojo. Or wear white after Labor Day. Consequently, I am kicked out of the Mushi-kera organization. I may or may not specifically be stripped of my sandan rank, given the rules of the school. But whether it is taken or not, that rank would be meaningless in any event since its value was only within the organization. True, I cannot be stripped of my physical ability and skills. But my rank would be moot. In other words, I am not, when I hold the rank, a sandan. I am a sandan *in the Mushi-kera school.*

Much the same is true for the license holder in a classical ryu who is kicked out of the ryu. He would still have his talents. But his license would have no value or meaning, since the authority that issued it has banished him. Being expelled from a classical ryu, incidentally, is relatively rare. The process is called *hamon.* It is extremely serious, something like being disowned from your family—which, in a way, it is. If you are expelled from a karate organization, there are dozens of others where you can begin your training again. In the very small world of the traditional martial ryu, however, people tend to know one another and word spreads fast. Unless you have a good explanation for your dismissal, it is unlikely you will be accepted into another ryu.

Both holders of dan-i and den-i ranks have also in common the matter of teaching authority. Neither a classical menkyo license nor a modern dan grade may necessarily be construed as permission to teach or to start one's own school or even start an authorized "branch" school. (In Japanese a branch school is usually called a *shibu.* The teacher there, who is instructing under the authority of either the headmaster or a representative, is the *shibu-cho.*) In some modern budo organizations, the rules may be that once you have reached a particular dan grade, you are automatically granted the right to teach. Some ryu licenses are explicit teaching licenses as well. In most cases, however, the recipient is, by tradition, also given oral permission by his teacher or the headmaster to actually instruct. Unfortunately, in some martial arts organizations, the "rules" about teaching are vague or nonexistent. A guy receives his black belt and assumes he now has mastered the art and opens his own school. Even if he is competent and even if his organization stipulates that once he reaches a certain grade he is able to teach, it is not necessarily a good idea. A budoka may be technically skilled but lack the personality to teach. This is an area where karate organizations have struggled. By not concentrating on teaching potential instructors *how* to teach, they have allowed incompetents into teaching positions, harming the quality and transmission of the school. If they were to regulate entry into teaching too tightly, on the other hand, they risk having potentially good instructors abandoning the organization in frustration. It will be interesting to see how martial arts groups continue to grow and change with regard to their ranking procedures and to see if they can improve on the old den-i methods of the feudal past.

21

THE "MARTIAL" IN A MARTIAL ARTS DOJO

I DON'T REALLY NEED to see a lot of your technique, your kata, your sparring or free-style exchanges, to know if you are training in a serious dojo. No experienced practitioner, in fact, needs to see much of that. Show me the dressing room at your dojo. That's enough.

Walk into the dressing rooms of some dojo and you will see clothes scattered everywhere. Bags and backpacks are on the floor. If there are training weapons used, the cases for them will be tossed here and there. Similarly, if there is a shoe box at the entrance to the place, the picture there will look the same: shoes piled haphazardly in a mound. Go into a serious dojo in Japan, and you will see an entirely different picture. (I do not mean to imply that every dojo in Japan is a serious one. Far from it.) There, you will usually find that clothes are hanging from hooks on the wall or folded and packed into the same bag the wearer brought his training uniform. Those bags are either hanging from hooks or placed on shelves or are stashed along a wall, out of the way. Footwear in the *kutsu-bako,* or "shoe-box," which is at the entrance of most dojo, is placed carefully. If shoes are left on the floor, they are paired neatly, the toes pointing toward the door so they can be slipped into quickly.

So is it that we are a nation of slobs and Japan is populated with neat freaks? Hardly. The average public toilet in Japan, by contrast, is far dirtier than those in the United States, for example. But there are two reasons for the distinction between the way many American dojo dressing rooms look and the way many of their Japanese versions do. The first is logistical. Japan is a small place. A population the size of the United States is living in space about equal to that of California. In such circumstances, people don't have the option to spread out. Once, when I was a young judoka, I was training at a university and getting dressed in the large locker room of the gym where the dojo was located. A Japanese senior to me came by and lectured me.

"Look at your clothes scattered all over the bench!" he admonished me. "Look how much space you're taking up!" I looked around. The locker room was huge. I was the only one in it. I didn't say anything, though. I recognized his point. From that time on, I began working to see how small a space my clothes and I could occupy when changing. Instead of tossing my clothes onto the bench or a chair and then dressing in my uniform, as I took my clothes off, I folded them. In old Japan, the dimensions of a tatami mat, about three feet by six feet, were considered adequate for a person to stand, sit, or sleep. I tried to change in half that space. It was a habit that proved valuable to have the first time I visited a Japanese dojo dressing room, where more than a dozen people were changing in a space not much bigger than a typical American bathroom.

The second reason Japanese dojo dressing rooms often appear neater is because their purpose was originally *martial*. We talk a lot about "martial arts." Too many times, though, we approach our training as if it begins when we bow into class and ends when we leave. If you are to seriously practice a budo, that isn't enough.

"Suppose you're training in the dojo and word comes that an enemy force is coming up the road," a sensei once told me. "You've got to either get yourself ready instantly or you've got to be able to run, to get away from the threat. How long is it going to take you to get your things and get into your shoes and get going?"

The answer to that question is the answer to why the serious dojo dressing room is arranged as it is. Now, of course we do not have to worry much about an enemy mounting an attack on our dojo. We *do* have to be ready for the unexpected—say, an earthquake or storm. The point, though, is that this is a *martial* place. We are training in a certain spirit, with a particular mentality.

It isn't just the dressing room in a Japanese dojo where you will see evidence of this mentality. One of the first martial lessons I learned was watching my sensei when we went into his house together. He took his shoes off at the door, then bent over and turned them around so they were facing out, away from the door. He didn't make a big deal of it. It was natural, like latching a gate shut once you'd passed through it. Anyone who's been to Japan will have seen that same gesture. Most of the people who do it there don't think about it, or, if they do, they just assume it is good manners they have learned as children. But the roots of this habit are in that sense of readiness, that extra moment that gets saved if you have to leave quickly—a moment that in the old days of Japan's long civil war could have been the difference between life and death.

In a traditional dojo, there are rules of etiquette for a wide range of activity. Which foot is used stepping into or out of the training area is prescribed. Look closely at this etiquette and in the majority of cases you will see that the "proper" way to do things is also the way that is most apt to keep you safe and prepared for an emergency.

Some will suggest this is just a fetish on my part, a preoccupation with seeing some martial intent in every Japanese custom or gesture. It isn't just Japanese, however. Military people have their own inculcated habits, traits they ingrain into their daily behavior, that can give them an edge. I know a former Special Forces officer who never wears pants without a belt. Even the shorts he wears in summer have loops with a belt threaded through. I asked him about it. Think of the advantage a belt gives you, he said. It can be a lifeline extended for someone to grab to pull them from a drowning situation. It can be used as a tie to handcuff a bad guy. A tourniquet. By making the wearing of a belt an everyday habit, the wearer gives himself an advantage in a wide range of emergencies. A fellow karateka and I were once sitting in an airport and watched a woman walking by in high heels and a skirt. He shook his head. "I never travel in clothes and shoes I can't run in, crawl in, or sleep in," he said. Good advice.

Approaching any budo as a sporting endeavor and nothing more, conducting oneself in the dojo as if one were in a gym: these lead a person away from developing these habits and attitudes. The budoka may enter the dojo and flop down on a couch in the entrance area for a while, then go to the dressing room and scatter his clothes or stuff them into a locker before getting into his uniform. If he isn't actively training, he may stand around, hands on his hips, talking, largely unaware of what is going on around him. He begins to focus only when he is engaged in training. Once the session is over, he resumes his casual attitude. For him, his art may be a great sport, a fine means of conditioning, or a great social activity. But it isn't really a martial art.

Please don't assume I am advocating a sort of paranoid, constant state of readiness where we might turn and break the jaw of a fellow dojo member who comes up and slaps us hello on the back. That kind of hypersensitivity is a caricature of the real martial spirit of readiness. Don't think of a rabbit in a field, constantly looking around, quivering, bolting at the slightest unexpected noise or movement. Think instead of a tiger—relaxed, calm, but always alert. The way to achieve this attitude is to pay attention to the little things and to incorporate a sense of awareness, not just in your training but in all aspects of your life. Looking around at your dojo dressing room is a good place to start.

22

DAILY LIFE FOR THE SAMURAI

WANT TO LIVE LIFE as a samurai would have? Want to follow the Way of the Japanese warrior? Okay. Pick up the sword. Tie on a headband. But first, get a degree in accounting.

Probably few images of the mysterious East have more attraction to Westerners than that of the noble samurai. Brandishing his razor-sharp *katana*, attired in flowing silk robes, composing elegant poetry, and dealing out death or meeting it with equal aplomb, he seems mythic. He is both stoic and sensitive. A hardened killer and a connoisseur of cherry blossoms scattering in the gentle wind. The samurai is a selfless paladin, ready to die at a moment's notice. He is an aesthete who forged himself like his perfect blade, living a life of honor, loyalty, and derring-do. This image of the classical warrior is invoked almost constantly in the Japanese martial arts. The noble samurai is, according to many martial artists, supposed to be our ideal, our model, our spiritual ancestor. We who train in the dojo today are "modern samurai," goes the story, the inheritors of a glorious, romantic, and bloody past. Or at least many might like to imagine. Of course, if you wish to pursue this notion, you are free to do so. You ought, however, to take a little closer look at that image before you buy too deeply into it.

To begin, talking about the samurai in general terms is like talking about an "American fighting man." That could be a reference to

111

anyone from a nineteenth-century Apache warrior to a Civil War soldier to a Vietnam-era Green Beret. Similarly, the samurai as a caste and as a political and cultural force developed over a period of almost one thousand years in Japan. There were moments in history when Japan had samurai who barely knew which end of the sword to hold; they were more at home playing party games and flirting than striding across a battlefield. At some times in Japanese history, the samurai class was one rigidly fixed by law. It was a hereditary title. A nonsamurai could no more have achieved that status than a peasant in Europe could have become a lord. At other periods, commoners like farmers or stable workers could and did become samurai. For most of us, the samurai is an iconic figure from one of two historical periods. He is often the warrior individual we associate with the Sengoku Jidai, the "Age of Warring Provinces." This was Japan's multifactioned civil war, lasting approximately from the fourteenth century through the start of the seventeenth. Our other common image of the samurai is from the later period of feudalism that finally ended in the mid-nineteenth century in Japan. This samurai is the hero of Akira Kurosawa movies: the stoic, taciturn warrior embodied by Mifune Toshiro, the lone hero brandishing his sword in the midst of battle, calm, composed—deadly. He is the Japanese version of the Western gunfighter, a loner, a drifting *ronin*—a masterless samurai—often, striding off into the sunset with a pile of bodies left behind him.

In historical reality, the samurai during this long period of feudal Japanese history were, in effect, members of privately maintained armies. Several daimyo, Japan's feudal lords, had by that era in Japan's civilization (the fourteenth century), amassed enough wealth and power to afford—and need—men who could defend and help enlarge the property and power of those lords. The stereotype of these daimyo that has emerged from this scenario is like some kind of James Bond–worthy villain, envisaged as the powerful lord who oversees his personal army, men-at-arms who spend their days constantly polishing their martial skills—or applying them in combat.

It is a cool picture. But look closer. Who pays for all the food those samurai eat? Who supplies their health care? Who provides clothing for them? And who foots the bills for all their spouses and children? The cost of supporting even half a dozen samurai and their families would have been ruinous, just as it would be today. Even the wealthiest daimyo would have gone bankrupt trying to keep up with the expenses of a squadron of warriors who did nothing but practice and employ their fighting arts.

The reality of the samurai's daily life is a little more mundane than the popular image. Actually, make that a *lot* more mundane. In addition to waging wars of conquest or protecting his assets, the daimyo had to concern himself with the more pedestrian realities of life. Taxes had to be levied and collected. Roads had to be built and maintained. Inventories had to be kept. These tasks fell to the samurai class. Formal education for the samurai was of considerable importance. Buddhist temples maintained early schools for the children of the samurai class. Later, Confucian-based academies were instituted in most fiefs. By the Edo period (1600–1867), these academies were under the control of the Tokugawa shogun who ruled the entire country. Classes in classical literature, along with those in science, mathematics, and ethics, were compulsory for the male children of the samurai caste in many fiefs. The well-educated samurai, then, were perfectly suited for employment as auditors, tax collectors, civil engineers, and for other clerical duties. That's how they earned their keep. The famous swordslinger Miyamoto Musashi was an engineer who designed and built several fortifications and castles. He was employed, in fact, by the Hosokawa clan, not as a swordsman or martial arts instructor but as an engineer. Given the enormous economic complexity of running a fief, a great many samurai earned their keep by keeping financial records and balancing the books. The samurai of the sixteenth century would have had much to talk about with today's Special Forces military. Chances are, he'd have had just as much in common with your local tax accountant or payroll clerk.

It might be a bit jarring, reconciling this reality with our idealized picture of Musashi, the solitary warrior-aesthete wandering about Japan, seeking duels in his quest for enlightenment: Musashi standing around, holding the feudal equivalent of clipboard, crunching numbers? What about the code of bushido that he and others were supposed to exemplify? A term that might be more commonly used in the West than in Japan, *bushido*, or "the way of the warrior," gained currency as the result of a book published in 1900 by Inazo Nitobe. Nitobe, a Japanese Christian, an economist, and a wonderful writer, attempted to explain the life and ethical pillars of Japan's warrior past to Western readers. Nitobe depended upon making equivalents he knew would be familiar to those readers: he drew from Greek and Roman history and from European chivalry. Well-meant and elegantly written, the book also unfortunately inculcated a number of misconceptions. Many of these arose because of the equivalents Nitobe and others who followed him tried to draw in an effort to make things more explicable to the West.

It is tempting to find a convenient drawer into which we might stick All Things Samurai. We can toss them in the drawer and know exactly what they all mean. "Bushido," especially after Nitobe's work was published, became that drawer. Trouble is, not every action or philosophy of the samurai fits so neatly into that drawer. Yes, for instance, a sense of loyalty to one's family was important to the samurai. Consider the case of the warlord Toyotomi Hideyoshi, however, who first named his nephew Toyotomi Hidetsugu as his successor. When Hideyoshi had a son, he changed his mind. Actually, that is putting it mildly. Hideyoshi exiled his nephew, then ordered him to commit suicide and demanded all of Hidetsugu's household do the same. When they were slow about it, Hideyoshi had all of them, including more than thirty women and children, murdered. Nagatoki Ogasawara, whose family name is among the best known of the warrior clans of Japan, was assassinated by his own samurai. Oda Nobunaga, was killed when one of his most trusted generals, Akechi Mitsuhide, turned on him. The great general Takeda Shingen got his start when he double-crossed his own father, having the elder Takeda taken as a captive by Shingen's father-in-law. There are many tales of samurai heroics. There are also tales of treachery and deceit. If we are going to consider bushido as the samurai's "code," we have to agree it is a very broad one, a code that seems to extol both loyalty and the most blatant perfidy.

Very broadly speaking, the samurai—and all of Japanese society from the fourteenth to the nineteenth century—were strongly influenced by Confucian philosophy. More precisely, it was the neo-Confucian scholar Chu Hsi whose version of Confucian thought became a guiding policy for the Tokugawa shogun who ruled Japan. A recognition of one's "place in life," articulated through relationships with others above and below one's station, was a unifying principle of this philosophy. From Chu Hsi's thoughts came many of the ideas of loyalty and service we think of in the samurai mentality. Yet in short, despite literature like Nitobe's book, there is no "code" to which the samurai universally subscribed. To insist there is a "samurai way" of doing things in the dojo or in life is simplistic and usually self-serving. If you are told, for example, that being ordered about by seniors in your dojo is a legacy of "bushido," you ought to laugh. The average Japanese today knows as much about the realities of life during the day of the samurai as you do about everyday life on the eighteenth-century frontier. Japanese and Westerners alike who cite the "samurai way" are usually misinformed or trying to justify their actions by appealing to a supposedly ancient code of conduct.

Another staple of the popular image of the Japanese warrior was *kiri-sute gomen,* the legal right afforded the samurai to kill commoners for any reason. A peasant didn't bow low enough as you passed by? Off with his head. *Tsuji-kiri,* or "cutting at the crossroads," describes killing a passerby if for no other reason than to test the quality of a blade. Yes, the samurai caste did have this right through much of the feudal period. And what happened when the right of *tsuji-kiri* was actually exercised? Say you beheaded that peasant for his insolence. The peasant, however, belonged to someone. He was part of the property of the local lord. He paid taxes, produced goods. Your killing just deprived the lord of those assets. Just as you, as a samurai, had the right to kill, the lord had rights as well. Your house, your property, even your position could be lost as the result of your actions. In truth, while samurai had the right to kill a commoner for any reason, they were also mostly smart enough not to indulge in it. It is interesting to note, as well, that the samurai and the commoners, particularly farmers, met in a number of armed conflicts. Usually these were started because of revolts over taxes. Samurai armed with sword, spear, and bow met mobs of farmers carrying axes, rakes, and rocks. And in literally every confrontation of this nature, the samurai lost.

Should we assume that because the professional warrior lost in pitched battles against farmers that his martial skills have been hyped and exaggerated? To some extent. One would, however, be mistaken in inferring that the samurai were not skilled and talented in combat. They did poorly against the farmer for the same reason the British did poorly at Lexington and Concord. They were faced with an enemy that fought differently, an enemy that presented political problems as well. Had samurai, defending against protesting farmers, slaughtered those farmers, the repercussions, politically and economically, would have been significant.

Think about it: the samurai would have been killing the source of their own food. Within the parameters of combat against other professional warriors, however, the samurai was, throughout much of his era as a distinctive class, successful. Even if we strip away all the tall tales and grandiose claims of lethality on the battlefield, the evidence that the samurai were an impressive military force is clear. However, we would do well to remember that grand victories in battle are but a very small component of what daily life was like for the classical Japanese warrior during a war or conflict.

One of my budo teachers has a scroll, one compiled by at least four generations of men in his family who have fought, participated in battles; men who came from a long line of samurai. The scroll is a collection of writings, filled with odd notes and bits of wisdom for dealing with daily life while engaged in military campaigns of the sort that were frequent during the feudal period. There isn't anything in the scroll about secret sword cuts that are invincible, none of the sort of "how to kill efficiently" stuff you might think. Instead, the scroll has recipes, like a concoction mixed to keep lice out of one's armor, and advice, like how to avoid food poisoning while eating the bacteria-laden fare that was often the diet of the man-at-arms in those days.

Look, war doesn't change much. It is miserable: hours and days of waiting to go into action, worrying, stewing, anxious and fearful. It is wearing the same, filthy, sweat-stained clothes weeks on end. It is being dehydrated, nauseated and weak from dysentery from drinking contaminated water. It is being sick with anxiety about families and work left behind. Under these conditions, just having enough strength to run across a battlefield would have been a nearly superhuman feat. Dreams of warriors are not about great victories so much as they are about a good night's sleep without being bitten by the bugs that have taken up residence in the crevices of your armor. In light of these conditions, the stunts that are the staple today of movies and other theatrical presentations about the samurai are simply comical: Leaping into the air to kick simultaneously at a pair of approaching enemies while cutting down a third? Doing cartwheels to escape an attack? Performing intricate cuts that require the precision of a surgeon? These skills are de rigueur in samurai and martial arts movies, but they have little to do with the combat reality for the fifteenth- or sixteenth-century warrior in Japan. That's why most older classical schools of martial arts involving weapons or grappling are demonstrably simple in their curriculum. True, often these schools will involve kata sequences and other training methods that are long and intricate, elaborate exchanges of attack and defense. To a considerable degree, these kata are for the purposes of improving cardiovascular fitness and endurance. Boiled down to their essence, the arts of the samurai intended for battle were practical, devoid of even the slightest unnecessary complexity. They depended on exquisite timing, or a willingness to come into the path of an attack before thwarting it, or some other principles difficult to acquire. But in terms of technique, they were simple. Modern combat methods often stress the same point—and largely for the same reason. Humans, under the incredible stresses of life-and-death combat, don't have to be lectured on the KISS principle ("Keep It Simple, Stupid"). They're living it.

You will sometimes see martial arts purporting a classical heritage that have fantastic, complex explanations for what they do. "Yes, if you strike between the third and forth intercostal regions at precisely a forty-five-degree angle, the opponent will suffer a rapid decrease in blood pressure and internal bleeding in the liver." Okay. Perhaps. Given the stress of close-quarters fighting, though, these sorts of pinpoint complexities have more application in the theory arena than in battle. Again, simplicity was the key.

Another standby of samurai movies is the revenge motive. A samurai takes off on an epic journey to avenge the slaying of his father or some other related figure. He wanders the countryside, looking for the killers, finally tracking them down and meting out justice with his trusty blade. As with the images of the vast private army doing nothing but training and fighting, it is an appealing picture. Again, who is paying for it? Samurai, remember, had jobs. They were bound, both by law and by loyalty and by financial commitment, to their lord. If you go to your boss tomorrow and tell him that you will be taking a year or two off to hunt down the killers of your family, he might be sympathetic. Or he might think you're nuts. Either way, he is very unlikely to say, "Okay, I'll be happy to pay your salary while you're gone. Where shall I send the checks?"

As with much of everything else in daily life in Japan, there were official rules of conduct on the matter of taking revenge for a killing. The first order of business for a samurai seeking revenge? Well, it wasn't to have your sword sharpened. No, it was to fill out the proper forms. You went to a magistrate and requested leave from your job.

There were regulations for taking revenge. If your father was killed, you might be granted permission and given a period in which your salary would be paid to your family. If it was an uncle, permission might be denied. Children were usually given permission to take revenge for the death of a parent. Parents, on the other hand, were often prohibited from doing the same for children. And those samurai who just quit, abandoned their lords on a quest of revenge? They would have had their homes and property seized by their lord, just as our houses would be eventually taken by the bank if we abandoned them. After they finished their quest for justice, such samurai would have often had difficulty finding employment later on. They would have faced, in other words, the same problems we would have today.

As we mentioned in an earlier chapter, in dojo all over the world, karateka are shouting "Osu!!" right now. In an aikido dojo, an instructor is walking around the class, pausing to give specific instruction to a pair of practitioners, and as he does, other training partners around him drop to kneel in respect to watch and listen. Once again, these practitioners may believe they are doing such things in the spirit of the samurai. More likely, they are doing things in the spirit of a U.S. military boot camp.

It was time for the lunch break at a seminar in the basics of Japanese swordwork that I gave not long ago, and as we all changed clothes, one intense young attendee walked into the hallway of the university that was hosting the seminar. He sat in a cross-legged posture more appropriate to yoga than budo, laid his wooden sword across his knees, and stared at the floor. I asked him to join us for lunch. "No thank you, sir." He was still sitting there when we returned. I learned later he was a student of a "master" who had concocted a fake ryu (largely from reading books and watching samurai movies) that demanded such relentless intensity. The teacher, and so his students, are really more caricatures of the classical warrior. For a real samurai, eating and relaxing were as essential as they are today. Adopting an attitude of a coiled spring works for a while. After a time, though, the tightly wound spring loses its flex. The energy is drained. The constant "at ready" mentality is the mark of an amateur, not a professional warrior. So it was for the samurai. At many times during the feudal period, warfare and the threat of violence were indeed daily concerns for the warrior class in Japan. They dealt with this in various ways, which included involving themselves in artistic enterprises like the tea ceremony or painting, and by indulging in drinking and attending parties and all the other distractions we know in our own era. They handled the daily stress in different ways. They were not, they could not have been, constantly coiled, their attention set on a hair trigger, engaged in the sort of stiff, artificial mentality we sometimes see today in dojo that confuse "militaristic" with "martial."

The Western notion of the military is very different from that of the feudal samurai's. Very few families in the West spawn generations of professional soldiers. The samurai were, for much of their existence, just that, a class of fighting men. Even in periods of peace, even if they were farmers or accountants or tax collectors, they came from a martial culture. They were literally born into it. When they began training in the martial arts, they did not need to be told how to behave in the dojo or training area. They knew the basics of handling a weapon. They knew how to obey orders. There was no need for excessive "militarism" in the training area.

A good analogy here is a comparison between the basic military boot camp and the training classes for Special Forces groups. In the former, one must contend with people who have no idea of how a military unit works, people who come from a civilian way of life. They have to acquire a certain mindset to be successful as part of a military unit. This is accomplished by drill, by going through every action of daily life, including just standing, according to a rigid form. Lots of shouting and intimidation. By the time a soldier is considered for Special Forces duty, however, he has been through all that. The classes in Special Forces training tend to be much more relaxed and informal. The intensity is still there. But now it comes not from authoritarianism on the part of the instructors or commanders. It comes from within the soldier. The samurai were in much the same position. Their legacy, their world, was one where martial activity was a standard part. The training in a dojo for the classical martial arts that are still surviving is typically relaxed. The alertness is natural, not contrived. Modern dojo that adopt a stiff, excessively formal atmosphere are actually demonstrating how far removed from the samurai mentality they really are.

The proliferation of video games set in mythic Japan, along with comic-book novels and movies, have contributed to images of the samurai that are almost absurdly romantic. Samurai are often depicted, for instance, with long, flowing hair. Japanese historical consultants in the movie *Shogun* insisted that the actor Mifune Toshiro, playing the lead Japanese role, should shave his head. The American director prevailed; he felt a bald samurai would not be attractive to Western audiences. He was probably right. From a historical perspective, however, the consultants were correct. Most of the renowned samurai of the feudal period shaved their heads. (It made wearing some kinds of armored headgear more comfortable and again, it acted as a way to prevent lice or other parasites from taking up residence.)

Another popular image of the samurai is an overlay of the Western template of the lone cowboy. Indeed, the notion of the wandering ronin, or masterless samurai, is so attractive many budo schools have named themselves "Ronin Dojo." That's odd. The most accurate translation of *ronin* is "homeless loser." Samurai who were good at their jobs, both in combat and as educated employees of a lord, didn't have much trouble finding employment. Very, very few samurai would have willingly adopted the life of the ronin. To a large degree, the samurai, like all members of feudal Japanese society (and to a considerable extent in modern Japan), identified himself within the context of those around him. Your proof of your worth was evidenced by how well you worked and fit into the group. Premodern Japanese society was communal in many ways. Individualism, as we understand it, is a Western idea. The solitary samurai, wandering off into the sunset in search of his destiny, is an appealing figure for us in the modern age. For the feudal Japanese, it would have been tragic and sad. A samurai's destiny was not in the sunset. It was among his comrades, with his family, serving his lord until his final breath.

Of course, our romanticization of those in the past is not confined to the samurai. We celebrate the cowboy, the medieval knight, the American Indian, as well. In these instances, however, our rosy view of the past is mitigated by abundant scholarship easily available and by the fact these figures are a part of our civilization. The very foreignness of the samurai makes them more exotic, less accessible, more subject to misinterpretation. It has long been an approach the West has had to Japan. We have the bare outlines of the samurai, or the geisha, and we color them in in a way that suits us, that satisfies our images of them. We think of the samurai as we would like them to be (or as we'd like to be them) and not, in many cases, as how they really were. To be sure, there were many samurai who were remarkable people. They accomplished extraordinary things. More than a century after they disappeared as a class, they continue to exert powerful influences on Japan. They have an influence on those of us in the dojo. If we really want to honor their proud legacy, however, we should do so not with silly, cartoonish caricatures more appealing to adolescents than to mature adults. We should study and read and discover who they really were.

Part Three

REFLECTING ON THE WAY

23

OKAY, NOW WHAT?

"How did you get started in martial arts?" This is a question
most budoka are asked, sooner or later. The Japanese martial Ways
have come more and more into the mainstream of American life
over the past half century. For many young people, enrolling in a
karate class is no more unusual than signing up to play little league
baseball or go to piano lessons. Most universities have judo or aikido
clubs. Even kendo is present in most big American cities. Still, it's
a little unusual, and those who know about your involvement are
often curious about what drew you to these budo.

One of my seniors notes that no matter how we explain it, the
reason at the heart of it, for virtually all of us engaged in the martial
arts, is fear. We are, at some time in our lives, afraid. We are afraid
of threats that might be made against us, of violence itself, of our
inability to handle stressful situations. We are fearful of our inadequacies, real and imagined. The budo are seen as a logical and reasonable response to those fears.

Once we are in the dojo we are confronted directly with our fears.
If I am frightened about the possibility of someone out there who
can beat me up, it is a dramatic confrontation to be in a room full
of people who undoubtedly *can* do that and who are, in a definitive
way, demonstrating their power to do so. Sitting in a library, I might

be able to convince myself I'm about as tough as those around me. Going to a judo dojo for the first time, it's a little harder to make that argument, even to myself. Once there, the process of my confrontation with my fears begins. A good teacher recognizes the element of fear as a motivation in beginners. We tend to think of fear as something we can get rid of, like ridding our house of cockroaches. We learn through a committed pursuit of budo that fear is more like the electrical wiring in our house. It's fundamental and it isn't going anywhere and while it can be harmful it is actually useful and can be put to good ends if we learn to use it properly.

Unfortunately, there are some—too many—in the dojo who never make it to that stage. They can never reach the point where they accept the fear, never learn to use it and, more important, to put it in perspective. These are often fanatically driven people. They are rarely happy people. Or mature people. Children worry about their self-image, their ability to compete. Most of them grow out of this. For those who do not—well, frankly, there's something a bit sad about a forty-five-year-old man who gets up every morning and looks in the mirror and wonders if he's still the toughest guy on the block.

When I come across these sorts, I always wonder what it is they wish for. What is it that continues to bring them to the dojo? I wonder what they would do if they could actually attain what they seem most to want. Consider this, if you are one of those people or if you know someone who is: Let's say you *are* indeed the toughest guy on the block. Toughest guy in the whole neighborhood, in fact. In fact, you've got the skills to clear a room of Israeli commandos without breaking a sweat. For all practical purposes, you are one invincibly good *bad* piece of work. Nobody's messing with you, and if they did, they would soon regret it. And so, now what?

In my imagination I can see these people reacting much like the country dog that chases every car that comes down the road, on that day when he actually catches one. What's he do with it? I do not mean to be dismissive of these people. Or to underestimate the reality of violence in our society today. But I do wonder about their sense of perspective. I often see fighting arts schools that play to the sense of fear in prospective students and that manipulate this perspective. They do not phrase it this way, of course. They are subtler. They will, they advertise, teach you "real-life combat skills." "Realistic self-defense." "We don't spend time on philosophy or religion," they typically explain. The implication, sometimes explicitly stated, is that such concerns are outside the realm of "real" fighting and self-defense.

We have, of course, flesh-and-blood examples of those individuals who did come very close to that extreme I have imagined. They did reach a stage where, while not invincible, they had power and skill that were awesome—so intimidating that few would have dared giving them a try in combat. By the early part of the seventeenth century, Yagyu Munenori was about as powerful as a martial artist could hope to be. The headmaster of the Shinkage ryu, his school was one of two chosen by the Tokugawa family as the official school of martial arts for the shogun. Munenori had accomplished the stuff of legend: In the Summer Battle of Osaka in 1615, Munenori led a contingent charged with protecting the Tokugawa shogun Hidetada. Unexpectedly during the battle, a group of warriors fighting for the Toyotomi broke from the woods, recognized Hidetada, and charged him. Munenori cut down seven of them, scattering the rest, saving the life of the shogun in a feat of swordsmanship that was extraordinary by any reckoning. Sure, in samurai movies, this happens to a warrior two or three times before he sits down to breakfast. In reality, facing multiple opponents successfully and killing seven of them is a feat so remarkable we would be tempted to dismiss it as fantasy had there not been several witnesses. Munenori was, by any definition, one tough hombre.

Munenori did not reach his position by political wrangling or bluster or a puffed-up résumé. He'd killed men, multiple enemies, in combat. His swordsmanship was at a frightening level. Certainly there are soldiers and others today who have killed as many, and more, as part of their duty or their job. But killing a person up close and bloody, killing someone with a blade, is different from shooting them from a distance. Munenori reached a place in terms of his skill and his experiences in combat that few have ever equaled. He must have had a glimpse, at least, of that place to which a lot of people seem to want to go: a kind of perfection of combat skill. And what did he see? I don't know, of course. I don't ever want to find out. But I think he looked into a blackness that must have been awful. I think he recognized that technical skills have their limit. I think, based on his history and his writing, Munenori understood that without some philosophical underpinnings, without a sense of morality and spirituality, combat skills have about them a destructive force that can take a person down a very dark path.

In Hotoku-ji, a small Buddhist temple in the village named after his family, there is a wooden statue of Munenori. He sits, wearing the vestments of a priest. The statue is extraordinary. What catches one's attention, however, is the gaze. Munenori's eyes peer out. Ebony, obdurate, they appear not focused on anything in particular, yet seeing all. This is the "gaze of the dragonfly," which Munenori wrote of in some of the texts he left for succeeding generations, a gaze that does not look at the predator bird hunting it but that, nevertheless, sees it and avoids the bird's attack. The manner of the dragonfly's gaze is considered a secret teaching in Munenori's ryu. Within the eyes of that statue of Munenori, I glimpse something of the spirit of a warrior. I see a man remarkably capable and skilled. There is a quiet determination in his eyes. He prevailed in combat. He prevailed in the cutthroat politics of his era, bringing success and security to his family and playing a fundamental role in the establishment of a school that would last many, many generations into the future. There is something else in that look as well, however. Maybe what I am seeing in those eyes is what so many others and I search for in our training: humanity.

There is much to be said about the need for self-protection in our world today. There is much to be said about the vast array of systems we have developed, modern and ancient, for dealing with the up-close violence we can encounter. I wonder though, if there is no more to be said about the value of our humanity in this context as well. After we've learned to defeat every possible enemy, control every possible threat, we must confront one more challenge: the challenge to be human.

24

CHOOSING A SENSEI

CHOOSING A SENSEI? I would start by considering what I do *not* want.

I do not want a daddy. I have had one. I do not need someone to love me and give me affirmation, someone I can idealize as a perfect, infallible role model and try to please. Instead, I want a person who can technically relay a budo's methods and who, by example, imparts the character of the art, its traditions and its values. I do not want a combination Yoda–Mr. Miyagi who is infinitely wise and can solve all my problems. I don't want someone who is living in a cave, metaphorically or literally, and who speaks in aphorisms and pseudo-"Oriental" platitudes. I have seen teachers who fancy themselves modern-day hermits or ascetics, living like monks. That is their right. But the Japanese budo were not meant to be practiced by those living on the fringes of society. They are meant to make us more productive and contributing members to society.

I do not want a sensei who is a budo teacher only because he isn't qualified—in terms of his formal education, his skills, or his ambitions—to be anything else.

I do not want a sensei who is not at least somewhat familiar with Japanese or Okinawan culture and who cannot pronounce Japanese with some proficiency. Many will disagree with me on this.

My teacher is not Japanese, they say. He is not living in Japan. Not teaching Japanese students. What does familiarity with the Japanese language or culture have to do with teaching karate under such circumstances? By way of answer, think of it like this: you wish to learn French cooking. You can learn from a chef who has spent time in France, speaks French, is conversant in French culture. He understands something of the civilization within which French cooking evolved. Conversely, you can apprentice with someone who claims to be an authority on French cooking but who can't pronounce a word of French, has never even visited that country, and who is clueless about French culture. Whom would you choose? It is unreasonable to expect every budo sensei to be an authority on Japan and fluent in Japanese. But they are, after all, teaching *Japanese* budo. A study of that art will always be more thorough and broader in perspective when it is taught by a person who has additional knowledge and understanding of the place where that art originated. The other day I had a conversation with a *rokudan,* a sixth-degree black belt in judo. He was talking about one of his students getting "six upons in a row." I realized he meant *ippon,* a full point given in judo competition. Come on. You have devoted all that time and energy, trained long enough to have received an advanced rank, and you can't pronounce a simple word of common judo terminology correctly? If you don't care enough to learn something as basic as that, how thorough and precise a teacher will you be? I wouldn't know. I wouldn't have someone like that as my sensei.

I also don't want a sensei just *because* he is Japanese. The notion that only the Japanese can truly understand budo and can transmit its techniques and spirit is silly on the face of it. There are some extraordinarily gifted martial arts sensei out there who are no more Japanese than Limburger cheese. I would no more confine myself to a sensei based on his race than I would confine myself to friends based on the same standard.

I would look for consistency in a sensei. "I started in tae kwon do, then I switched to Goju ryu, then I did a little Brazilian jujutsu, but

I've been teaching Shito ryu now for about three years." To some, this may suggest a broad perspective in fighting arts. To me, it suggests a guy who can't commit to something and stick it out. Consistency applies as well in where you teach. There are teachers who seem to bounce around, teaching here and there. That's understandable to a degree. Space for training is expensive and hard to find. But when a teacher can't seem to keep a group together, can't keep a group large enough to support itself in terms of rent, I am suspicious.

I would look for reliability in a sensei. The sensei I have admired have been there, week after week, year after year, always in the dojo, training and teaching. Their students knew, coming to practice that night, that Sensei would be there. Consistently, they have taught their budo as it was taught to them. Fads come and go. Crime goes up, and some martial arts training halls institute special "self-defense" classes. A movie comes out featuring samurai, and karate dojo begin offering classes in "Japanese swordsmanship." I want a sensei who knows what his art is, knows its boundaries, and stays within them. Conversely, I want a sensei who isn't teaching robotically, unquestioningly. Many "ballistic" stretches and other training methods have proven to be unhealthy. A good sensei has discarded these, even if they were a part of his training in years past. The sensei worth following knows how to evaluate what he's doing and to change when necessary. He doesn't follow tradition for tradition's sake. He adapts. His goal is to use the tradition, not to be bound by it.

I would look for a sensei who is part of the community, one who has friends and relationships outside budo. I would want a sensei who is a good citizen and takes seriously his obligations to his family and his neighborhood and his country. I would want a sensei who is devoted to budo, not consumed by it, or worse, defined by it. I wouldn't want a sensei who happens to be a good person. What I would look for in a sensei is a good person who happens to teach budo.

Am I being naive in setting such standards for a sensei? Possibly. Am I going to find such a search challenging? Probably. Is it worth it? Absolutely.

25

WHAT IF?

IF THE SUBJECT WAS "the best karateka in modern times," how long would we be discussing it before the name of Hirokazu Kanazawa came up? To any serious martial artist, the name is instantly familiar and conjures a sense of respect that borders, especially to those who have seen him in person, on awe. Kanazawa, the chief of the Shotokan Karate International organization, is unquestionably one of the most skilled practitioners of that art alive. I cannot imagine my readers, even if their chosen budo is not karate, will not know of him. If not, briefly:

Kanazawa began his karate training with the Japan Karate Association after World War II. His seniors and teachers included Hidetaka Nishiyama, Teruyuki Okazaki, and Masatoshi Nakayama. In 1957, Kanazawa entered the All-Japan Karate Championships despite a broken hand and despite the fact he had never even trained in free-sparring for competition; he won. His tournament record has never been equaled. Kanazawa was among the first generation of karateka to graduate from the fabled JKA instructors training program. In the years since, he has taught karate on every populated continent in the world. He heads the Shotokan Karate International, overseeing the karate education of literally hundreds of thousands of karateka globally.

Kanazawa did not reach this level of expertise easily. During his early days of training he punched and kicked in endless repetition, day after day, year after year, until his body was reduced to a supple mass of sinewy armor. Today, training with him reveals, even in the simplest of his body movements, his extraordinary level of skill. He sometimes gives the impression that he is able to glide above the ground in fluid motion and then, at the focus of a technique, he looks to be rooted inseparably from it. The force of his kicks reverberate the air around him. Onlookers from yards away have been seen to flinch.

By any standards, Kanazawa sensei is a formidably powerful man. He possesses the physical strength for which our culture has always afforded respect. Just as famous athletes inspire their fans and followers, Kanazawa and the other budo experts who have taught and demonstrated here are a source of admiration and emulation for American martial artists. Those who have trained with sensei at Kanazawa's level will tell you that it is easy to become mesmerized by that kind of strength. They come to accept the idea that it is a strength that is, for all practical purposes, invincible. Yet Kanazawa and others like him are human. Kanazawa's reverse punch could crush my skull like an eggshell. As a defense against even a puny compact car traveling at seventy miles an hour, however, and hitting Kanazawa in a crosswalk? The punch wouldn't do much. Kanazawa can block your roundhouse kick so powerfully it feels like your foot's come in contact with a cattle prod. But his blocks against the attack that muscular dystrophy could launch against his body tomorrow would accomplish little more than one put up by your grandmother. The point is that Kanazawa and every other great martial artist is subject to accidents or illnesses just like the rest of us, misfortunes that could, in an eyeblink, destroy every last bit of his legendary strength. What if that did happen? It might be awful but still worthwhile to reflect upon that question. Where then would Kanazawa—or any of the rest of us—be?

If Kanazawa's strength had been built through weight lifting or conventional athletic endeavor, its loss would result in his fading away, no doubt, becoming one of yesterday's soon-forgotten celebrities. Perhaps, as some in the field of sports have done, he would try embarrassingly to maintain a facade of competence in an invariably doomed attempt to stay in the eye of his followers. Or, he might become bitter and morose over the fate dealt him, withdrawing into drugs or alcohol. Even if he were able to handle the emotional disaster of a serious physical impairment, if Kanazawa had been trained as an ordinary athlete, he would have joined the ranks of those sportsmen who lives are forever and tragically reduced by their inability to practice and perform.

Traditional karate training, however, like all budo training, does not follow the same regimen as that of sports. Nor are its goals similar. Oh yes, karateka, just like all budoka, try very hard to make their muscles more efficient, to improve their cardiovascular endurance; in short, they work just like any athlete to be stronger. But far more important to the martial artist is the development of a different kind of strength, one that does not depend so much on the physical as it does on the spiritual. This kind of inner strength is what we might refer to as *damashi*.

Budo no damashi, the "spirit of the martial Ways," is something that transcends the limited capabilities of the body. It is that part of the budoka's personality not immediately evident. It is molded by those long hours practicing the art's basics, fortifying the spirit, and by the even longer hours spent learning advanced techniques that will take a decade of work before there is some kind of understanding of their movements. Damashi is nurtured by the courage necessary to face a vastly superior opponent in a match, with the hope not of winning but of gaining some insight from the encounter. It is a refined sort of toughness that cannot be acquired through the cursing of a drill sergeant or a football coach, or even through a teacher's instruction. Rather, damashi is an attribute attained through an intensely individual commitment to the martial Way, the ultimate aim of which is in the perfection of the self.

In talented and dedicated budoka, damashi is what eventually spills over from their practice in the dojo and influences their everyday life. It allows them to meet successfully the rigors, setbacks, and challenges of life with the same calm determination that they draw on to approach similar experiences in their training.

Damashi is a subtle strength. It is really discernible perhaps, only to more advanced students of the martial Ways who have at least started on their own journey toward making damashi a part of their own character. Even so, damashi is one of the vital elements that distinguishes the budo from sport or entertainment. Its presence is one characteristic that distinguishes the budoka from the athlete. Patiently developed as a part of serious training and long, long commitment to an art, damashi is a kind of fortitude. Illness, injuries, the toll time takes on our bodies; any of these might prevent Kanazawa or any other budoka from ever getting out on the dojo floor and physically practicing their budo again. Life's uncertainties can take this from us. Even so, damashi allows Kanazawa and the rest of us who follow the Ways to continue on. We may remain worthwhile as human beings, stable of center, at peace with ourselves and with the rest of the world. Physical power and technique are transient. Grace and dignity are timeless. Damashi is the element that elevates budo in such a way that we can realize this and embody it.

The techniques of budo as performed by their greatest experts instill awe in the rest of us. Rightfully so. They should be observed at every opportunity, copied as faithfully as we can in our own practice. But budoka, especially those who are young and healthy and bursting with energy and enthusiasm, should never forget that physical skill and ability are tools. Those tools are important for building a body strong enough to practice budo. Yet energy and enthusiasm are even more important for creating the kind of damashi, the kind of spirit that will sustain those budoka long after an accident or illness or age has ebbed their strength.

The future of any young martial artist practicing today will certainly have a few clouds on its horizon. That is to be expected. Aikido's founder, Morihei Ueshiba, endured a series of illnesses that robbed him more than once of all the strength he had built up. Gichin Funakoshi lived through the misfortunes of a war that destroyed his dojo and many of his best students, including one son. Misery and suffering and loss are part of life. However, if training is steadfast and sincere, the spirit of today's budoka will carry them on as it did for martial artists of other times. That is the final purpose of budo's damashi.

26

DADDY HITS ME BECAUSE
HE LOVES ME

Have you ever been in a dojo where the training was so harsh you might have wondered if it was bordering on actual abuse? If so, I hope you did not stay. If you were wondering, chances are that your suspicions were correct. Unfortunately, there are dojo where physical abuse or other sadistic behavior is thinly disguised as "hard training."

I heard a young karateka on TV not long ago explain the way things work in his dojo. The teacher regularly selects a student for some "free-sparring," which is basically an opportunity for everyone else in the dojo to watch while the teacher beats the student. The TV program highlighted the sparring sessions. The guy was punched, full force, and kicked, swept to the floor repeatedly until he was crouched like an animal, sobbing. He was once hit so hard he confessed to the camera later that his rib might have cracked. But it was, the guy explained, all because Sensei wanted to toughen him up, to make him stronger. One could not help but think of the little kid, his eye swollen shut and purple, explaining that his father had done it but only "because he cares about me."

There was a lot of uncomfortable, nervous laughter among other students during this session. One sees the same sort of reaction among a group of onlookers when a bully is tormenting someone. The onlookers are afraid to confront the bully or protest his actions; their laughter is a way of deflecting their discomfort. However, given that the guy was a Caucasian, training in an Asian dojo, perhaps the laughter was genuine, a twisted pleasure taken in having the foreigner beaten up.

Of course, theoretically the student can hit back in these situations. Realistically, there are several reasons the student would not. He might not be at a technical level that would allow him to get his strikes in. Even if he was, there is a considerable intimidation factor in going all out and whaling on one's teacher or even in trying to. The budo, after all, constantly reinforce the status of the teacher. Even a good sensei has to deal with the reality that his presence can be intimidating to his students. A bad one uses that, psychologically, to bolster his status within his group.

Well, I will be told: This is the way it is in budo. I don't understand the "samurai way" that dictates a harsh, brutal training environment. Cry in the dojo and you will be victorious "on the street." Okay. If you are an adult and that's what you want, then I think you've got something really important missing in your emotional makeup, but you are free, of course, to do as you wish. None of my business. Claiming some kind of historical basis for this, however, is absurd. It is perpetuated by people who don't know much about what life was actually like for those samurai. We've explored this misunderstanding of life for the samurai in an earlier chapter. I would like to focus a little more narrowly for a moment here.

In today's military, especially those branches like the Special Forces, training is notoriously rigorous. It's tough. Trainees are often injured, and some die each year. Those who equate this with the training of the samurai in feudal Japan, however, miss a very basic point. What happens to those who can't cut it in the Army Ranger program, for instance? They wash out and return to the regular military. What happens to those who can't, for reasons physical or psychological, make it through the basics of Marine Corps training? They are, in most cases, given a discharge. Neither the Rangers nor the Marines are troubled by this: they have a steady supply of people who want to join and who will take the place of those who have left. In extreme cases where there might not be enough applicants, a draft can be instituted. But for the most part, there is a large pool of candidates willing to undergo severe training. It wasn't like that at all for the samurai.

Most fiefs in old Japan were comprised of very small populations. Japan's geography is not conducive to supporting a large population in an agrarian sense. The average daimyo would have been in control of a few thousand people at most. He did not have a huge pool of candidates, not for farming or for any other needed occupation, including that of military service. Further, villages and communities consisted of very tightly knit groups. Clan and family connections were close. A young man could not, under normal circumstances, "wash out" of military duties, not if he were a hereditary member of the samurai class or a conscripted soldier. Everyone had to pull his own weight; there was simply no excess of manpower. In a sense, those in charge of military matters within a fief had to use what they had, and what they had wasn't sufficient to allow them to pick and choose.

All of this is not to say that training in a martial art in old Japan was easy or as convivial as a neighborhood barbeque. Life pretty much everywhere on the planet was a lot tougher for everyone prior to modern times. The warrior class in Japan adhered to a certain stoic sensibility. One had to be able to accept pain and deprivation. In classical martial arts training today, which comes close to the training regimens of the samurai, injuries are not unheard of. I don't know of a single practitioner of a classical martial art who hasn't been injured. In nearly all cases, however, these injuries come because one is ramping up the level of intensity *after having learned the basics*. Sequences of techniques within a kata come faster and faster, the better one gets. The distancing of safety gets cut closer and closer. I have heard and seen (and actually experienced) a teacher accidentally injuring a senior student in the context of rigorous training. (I have, much more often, seen the teacher get hurt in these exchanges.) I have never seen a teacher, not in any serious way, accidentally or deliberately injure a beginner or a student from the junior ranks of his dojo. That's because safety must be a primary concern within traditional training. Whack a student before he has developed his skills and a perspective to deal with such physical contact and you risk losing him, either through a crippling injury or because he becomes intimidated, his spirit broken. If you have three hundred students studying with you, this loss may be acceptable. If you only have a dozen or so, that loss is going to be considerable for your dojo and your art. That was the reality for the samurai in his training.

The modern budo operate in a different paradigm than the classical combative arts, true. And if it is some "tradition" in your art or your dojo that students are beaten, again, that's your business. But please do not claim some ancient "samurai" source for such a tradition. It does not exist.

In any serious fighting art, the psychological and emotional development of a trainee must be given not just equal but actually greater emphasis than the physical element of training. Why? First, because the ability to maintain and deliver weapons to the target is at least as essential as having the weapon itself at hand. You can teach anyone to pull the trigger of an automatic rifle in moments. Teaching him to aim it under stress or difficult circumstances, to maintain it and repair it—these lessons take much longer. Second, while our bodies eventually reach a physical peak in terms of stamina and conditioning, our mental skills can continue to be refined. A sixty-year-old cannot kick as hard as a twenty-year-old, not in muscular terms. Nor can he exert the same kind of force in a throw or a locking technique. But well beyond the age of sixty, he can continue to develop the ability to read a situation, to psychologically "lead" an opponent so timing and mental control of the situation and other factors work to make his technique far more devastating than it might be in a younger person who has not refined such skills. Helping a student develop the confidence and mental acuity to polish and refine these more subtle talents requires a very sensitive teacher who can temper, through careful heating and cooling, the steel of a student's mind. You cannot simply take the raw iron ore, throw it in the fire, then beat it until a good steel emerges. You don't make quality that way. Not in steel, and not in a human in a dojo.

27

A LITTLE COMMON SENSE

PEOPLE, COME ON. Let's use just a little common sense, shall we?

I was just directed by a reader to a website devoted to a system of fighting that reader has studied for many years. The site is extensive, with long, detailed histories of the art. The art started—of course—in a secluded monastery. It was preserved in utter secrecy, inherited by a noble hero who left China after defeating an entire company of sword-wielding Japanese soldiers and who then showed up in Los Angeles in the early 1960s. It all sounded ever so romantic and exciting, except: the name of the art makes no sense in Chinese. The phonetics don't exist in any dialect of Chinese. It is like having an art you claim is American in origin that's written "fzzbkeqqt." Those letters can't even be pronounced in English. I asked the reader about this. He told me the master's American students couldn't pronounce the real name so the master changed it. Okay, so we are supposed to believe this teacher produced a couple of dozen "masters" who teach all over the country—but he couldn't instruct a single one of them to pronounce the name of his art?

Many years ago I read about a fellow, a teacher of some kind of Chinese fighting art, who had, he explained in the article, learned from a mysterious Chinese master named—more than three decades later I can still remember it—"Cat Clung Ling." Come on. All it would have taken was a trip to a Chinese restaurant or to some other place with native Chinese speakers, to inquire and discover than two of these three names do not occur in any Chinese dialect. True, that article was written a long time ago, back in the 1970s. Most Americans knew little about China, and one tends to trust one's teacher, no matter what the decade. But today, when you're fed a line it only requires a few clicks on a keyboard to check out some obvious parts of the tale. And an art or a name that do not grammatically or phonetically exist in the language where that art is supposed to have originated is a pretty good clue.

I like the arts that place their age at some exact moment in time, "1,500 years ago," but then go on to explain that the origins are lost in the mists of history. Yeah. Your art is older than the recorded history of that country, but you can't even name its leader before 1962. The *xia chao fan* forms you do are exactly like those taught in the Taoist monastery in far-off Kung Pao Province in the ancient LaChoy Dynasty. But uh, your teacher's teacher was somebody named Wing or Wong, and you don't know anything beyond that. It is interesting how some people's arts have detailed histories, anecdotes, and lore that date back centuries—the farther back in time, it often seems, the more detail is available. Ask these people about recent history, though, names and dates and places that might be more easily documented, and they start to mumble.

One famous art claims origins back to an era in Japan when the Japanese were still virtually in the Stone Age. For years, books were published and stories were told about the direct lineage of the art, dating right up to the current, incumbent grand master. Often at the center of these narratives was a figure from the early twentieth century, a direct link to the feudal past of this art. Finally, someone asked, "Hey, is there any evidence this guy even existed?"

It wasn't as though the fellow lived in the mists of the ancient past. Japan, at the beginning of the twentieth century, was a modern nation, with extensive record keeping. In some ways, the documentation was better and more complete than what we had at that time in the United States. Somehow, though, this mysterious master has slipped through the cracks of history, any evidence of his existence vanished. (To put this in perspective, imagine being unable to present a single shred of evidence of your great-grandfather. No records of military service, tax or census records, no newspaper obituary, no place where he ever worked.) Predictably, the practitioners of this art howl with outrage at any questions regarding this figure, challenging the motives of those who ask and insisting in the end that the story is simply too good *not* to be true. At times like this, one despairs. How can people embrace such obvious silliness?

Many of these far-fetched and ambitious tales came about during the late 1960s and early 1970s. A lot of readers today weren't even born then, so it may hard for them to understand just how little was known about Asia in general and the fighting arts of that part of the world in particular. We were talking earlier about unlikely and impossible names, for instance. Watch early episodes of the crime drama *Hawaii 5-0*. You'll hear bad guys with "Japanese" names like "Rashiri," which are about as Japanese as yogurt, and see Caucasian actors portraying Chinese with bad, absurdly crude makeup jobs. Very few people knew the difference between judo and karate; even fewer had ever heard of things like kung fu or kendo. In such a climate, misinformation was common. Outright fraud was difficult to detect. Today, most martial artists, by contrast, will have access at a college or cultural institute to a native speaker of Chinese or Japanese. They can check out a story or a document. If not, there are sites on the Internet where such things can be put out for inspection, and experts can easily and quickly explain what's right or wrong about it all.

Also—and this is important—not all practitioners of an art have an interest in its history and provenance. A person may think: My art is fun to do. It looks effective for what I want as a means of self-defense, or sport, or artistic endeavor. I don't need to know the name of my teacher's teacher's teacher to enjoy myself. I don't need to know in what province in Japan this art supposedly originated in the sixteenth century to benefit from practicing it. That's reasonable. However, if that is your approach, then you must be honest when questions are asked. You must acknowledge you don't know anything about the art's history. You can point those inquiring to information put out by your school. But you should not become angry or defensive when legitimate questions are asked about that information. If it is a story, handed down through your family, that one of your ancestors was a pivotal hero at Gettysburg but the veracity of that story matters little to you, that's fine. But you should admit, when a researcher questions the accuracy of your family's story, that it is only that, a tale told for which you have no proof and have never yourself researched.

Let's face it, there is romanticism and mystique regarding the martial arts and at least some of it has to do with the fabulous tales of the history and origins of these arts. Remember, though, these three things: One, just because your ancestor actually *was* a hero at Gettysburg doesn't mean anything at all about you. Living off the reflected glory of some heroic, mythic past is not admirable. Maybe the founder of your art did kill a dozen attackers single-handedly. That doesn't mean you have any special power or skill unless you get it the same way he did, by hard work and effort. Two, when legitimate questions are raised about the history or origins of your art, they are not necessarily personal attacks or even attacks on the efficacy of the art. Yes, you may have used techniques from the art to defend yourself successfully against a crazed SAS commando. That does not prove your art dates back a thousand years. And three, if you are interested in your art's history and are investigating it, come on. Use a little common sense.

28

"I DON'T NEED TO TRAIN ANYMORE"

YOU THINK YOU'VE HEARD IT ALL. You think that after a certain number of years being involved in the Japanese martial Ways, there's not much that can still surprise you. You are wrong. At least I was. I really could not believe what I was hearing.

A friend related the conversation, one he'd had while attending an open clinic presented by a visiting karate instructor. My friend was introduced to some other karateka at the seminar, people who let it be known very quickly to him that they were "seniors" and were, in fact, instructors themselves and very highly positioned in their organization. My friend noticed immediately as the seminar began that these people did not participate in the warm-up session. They didn't join in the training that followed. Instead, they stood at the front of the room and watched. During a break, my friend approached one of these people and asked if perhaps he would be joining in the training later on in the day.

"I don't train anymore," the fellow told him. He said the guy actually seemed surprised at the thought of training. "I'm a senior instructor," the fellow said. "I don't train anymore. I just teach."

As I said, I tend to be cynical in assuming I have heard it all. I am accustomed to being told stories of "tenth-degree black belts" who aren't old enough to remember the first Bush administration. Of masters so deadly they are enjoined from regular practice because their techniques are simply too dangerous to be exercised around mortals. But the notion that one can reach a level in karate where no further training is necessary? I must admit, I was speechless. Had I not known my friend well and respected his honesty, I'd have thought he was making it all up.

The idea that one can reach a point in karate or any of the budo—or any *do* form of traditional Japan: tea ceremony, flower arranging, whatever—is just so utterly preposterous it beggars the imagination. It is something like saying, "I am so good at marriage, I have perfected my marriage to such a degree that I no longer need to be married." We would laugh at the silliness of such a statement, right? Because becoming good at marriage, building and refining and keeping a marriage strong and healthy, is a lifelong process. You don't graduate from a "marriage academy," learning all that is needed and so becoming free of any further involvement. No, you must continue working, learning, and contributing to a marriage either until you or your spouse dies or until you are no longer married.

Let's be absolutely clear: There is no graduation from the budo. There is no summit, no peak you reach at which point you can say, "I've climbed to the top; there is no place higher for me to go." Instead, the path of a martial Way is like working your way slowly up a hill. It is not a steep or treacherous one. But if you have never climbed before, the path can look and feel intimidating. And it is deceptive. You approach the top—or at least what you believe to be the top—proud of your accomplishment. And then you see it. Once you have reached the summit, three or four larger hills loom up in front of you. Each of them must be climbed. When you climb the first, it affords you a view of half a dozen more peaks that are even higher. The second reveals another vista, of other peaks that are more like mountains. Each time you tackle a new climb, you are rewarded the same way. Another landscape, filled with more mountains. You cannot, in fact, imagine having the time or energy or resources in what remains of your life to climb even a fraction of those peaks you have glimpsed in the distance.

For some, this description of the pursuit of budo will seem familiar. And exciting and challenging. That a martial Way offers vistas and destinations so varied and profound they cannot be explored in a lifetime is a powerful attraction for these people. For others, I suppose, the view from the top of that first little hill is intimidating. There is something within these kinds of people, something small, some tiny voice from the depths of their ego that whispers to them. They turn their back on the hills and mountains. "I've reached the top!" they tell everyone, including themselves. And they hope others will believe them. And they hope too, I suppose, that they can believe it themselves. And they spend the rest of their lives not out conquering new summits but marching around and around the crest of that first little hill, reliving their accomplishment, pretending those higher elevations aren't out there.

To me, this is the only real explanation for someone to believe he no longer has a need to train in a martial art, that his efforts should not be in the pursuit of his own journey but rather in sitting comfortably and shouting instructions to those below. True, he can help those below climb to his position. He can help them climb no higher. Indeed, those who have climbed higher and who encounter a person of this sort realize instantly that he is deluding himself or others. My friend from that day at the seminar has climbed much higher. He has sought out teachers, made sacrifices, trained hard. He continues to train even though he is now teaching as well. He sees karate-do from a very different perspective from those sad characters standing at the front of the training hall and watching.

The great joy and the wonderful benefit of following a martial Way—please understand this—is in the *process*. That is a big reason it is called a martial Way. It is a path. It is not a destination. There are endless destinations along the Way. Some of us will reach more of these destinations than will others. In the end, what matters is not how many summits we climbed. The value of budo is in the process of spending our lives doing that climbing. Tomorrow I may be struck with an illness or an accident, as we noted in an earlier chapter. I may never be able to make a front kick or a hip throw or a strike with the sword ever again. You, who are still healthy and active, will keep on climbing and reach places I never see. Nevertheless, my training will not have been wasted. It wasn't spent, so far as budo goes, in getting somewhere. It was spent in the process of the trip itself.

Of course, there may be cases where physical limitations mean a budoka can no longer be active. If one of my teachers were confined to a wheelchair or had to walk with a cane, limiting his activity, I would still seek his teaching and guidance. And I do not mean to imply that once one reaches such limitations, through age or other debilitating factors, that his particular journey on the way of karate is over. In his final years, Gichin Funakoshi had to be carried up the stairs to get to the dojo where he taught. I suspect, however, that he was still struggling, still climbing some of the peaks of his art, even if these mountains were ones we still down in the lower peaks may know nothing about. Following a budo is as much mental and emotional and spiritual as it is physical. Age, illness, or injury, however, did not particularly reduce the so-called senior instructors at the seminar my friend attended. They were physically capable of movement and activity. That is what is so terribly sad about their attitude. A much older karate teacher once said to me, "By the time I got old enough to know how I was supposed to do it, I was too old to do it." These people were not that old, not that frail. Their limitations were not physical. Their limitations were in their own crippled egos.

The notion I am embarking on a journey I will never finish, that I am going into a place the dimensions and boundaries of which it is impossible fully to know, can be daunting. That is what we sign up for when we begin to follow the path of budo. An "instructor" who thinks otherwise? He will never be my instructor.

29

FOLLOWING THE WAY

A FELLOW WHO USED to come to the dojo, one who was very taken with the spiritual aspects he saw in the aikido we were training in there, told us once that it was okay for him to miss training because, as he put it, "Even when I'm playing my guitar, I'm practicing my aikido." We were patient with this guy, though he was, I admit, the butt of some jokes when he wasn't around—off polishing his throws, no doubt, by twanging the chords of "Stairway to Heaven." We weren't surprised, either, when he abandoned his aikido training. A great deal has been made in popular writing about how following a martial art will and should pervade other areas of our life. This has led to some silliness, as with believing that, just because you strive to approach it with the same intent and feeling, playing a guitar is the same thing as getting out on the dojo floor and training. The fact that my balance, improved through my aikido, allowed me to cross the swift current of a river while swimming last weekend does not mean a weekend playing in the river will improve my aikido.

Likewise, much has been made of the notion that all the traditional *do* of Japan—the budo, *shodo* (calligraphy), *kado* (flower arranging), and *chado* (tea ceremony)—are, at their core, similar: that they all share the same goals. While this is true, we must be careful not to draw far-fetched conclusions about it. There is a famous story told about a master of the tea ceremony who inadvertently insulted a samurai. The tea master was challenged to a duel; he had no choice but to accept. In desperation, the tea master went to an expert swordsman and explained the problem. "Make tea for me," the swordsman told him. The tea master did so, going through the ritual as though it might be his last—which it well could have been. "Exactly," the swordsman said. "Just approach the duel with the same spirit in which you made that tea." You know what happened, of course. The tea master appeared at the site for the duel so calm and composed, filled with the spirit of the tea ceremony, that the samurai lost courage and fled. Great story. And a worthy point. In reality, the tea master would have died. Spirit is wonderful. But it cannot replace technical skill. You want to become good at karate? Practice karate.

We would be foolish to believe an expert with the sword would automatically be able to pick up a brush and be a competent calligrapher, or that an expert in flower arranging, just because it shares a similar spirit with karate, could perform a great kata. However, we would be ignorant not to see the parallels between the various traditional *do* of Japan. Just as a visiting instructor or a trip to a seminar in another dojo can present some facet of your karate or any other budo in a different light, sometimes what's presented to us by those following other Ways can give us a different perspective on what we do.

Sen Soshitsu XIV was, as his title implies, the fourteenth headmaster of the Urasenke style of the tea ceremony. He headed the ryu during the critical time in Japan's history, from 1924 to 1964,when Japan emerged as a world power, was subsequently crushed during World War II, and was later rebuilt into a modern nation. It was Sen's idea to plant the tea ceremony in Western cultures, and he traveled to the United States and Europe to present it. Sen Soshitsu was writing about the tea ceremony, of course, in the following paragraph. Read his words, however. And when he writes about the Way of tea, think "martial arts" instead. When he writes about the "tea hut," think "dojo." And his references to "the spiritual taste of tea," translate that for yourself into the "spirit of budo." Please do that as you read this from the master's *Tea Life, Tea Mind* (Weatherhill):

> To those aspiring to follow the Way of Tea, guard against jealousy. Placing yourself at the center of things, envying or tempting others—these are unpardonable. Know your duty, and immerse yourself daily in the Way of Tea and you will find contentment. The more you look up to others, the clearer your own position in relation to them will be. Whenever something bad happens, people try to make themselves look as good as possible. But if we remember the humility of the host in the tearoom, someone who knows the spiritual taste of tea, then this constant craving of power for its own sake will be seen for what it is. Know what you know and know what you don't know, for only then will the limits of your strength become evident. To attain spiritual power, seize the chance when it offers itself; devote yourself to study and practice. In life are many who feign knowledge and lead others astray. No action can be more reprehensible. The Way is never exclusive. It is open to all to follow, but those who set out upon the path perforce need the way of those who have passed that way before.

Okay, you tell me: did this master of the tea ceremony have anything to say that is of value to budoka? Sen Soshitsu did practice martial arts, by the way. He practiced both judo and kendo, back in the days when those arts were a lot closer to combat than they were to sports. Physically, he was a powerful man. But he never practiced budo at the level where you and I are practicing it. His duties as headmaster of a tea school would have prevented it, even if he had wanted to. Sen Soshitsu was a guy who practiced the tea ceremony all day long. I don't think he could have shattered a stack of boards with his tea scoop. I doubt he could have used it as a weapon for self-defense against an attacker. So perhaps it is reasonable to conclude he couldn't possibly add anything worthwhile to the education of a budoka.

"Placing yourself at the center of things," being jealous of others, trying to look good when things go wrong—these are flaws he was addressing in *chadoka,* or exponents of the tea ceremony, not karate or judo. When he advises to remember the importance of humility and to avoid "craving power for its own sake," that was meant to be applied in the tea hut, not the kendo or aikido dojo. Knowing how much you don't know in order to appreciate and expand the limits of your own strength—surely there isn't a lesson in those words for the budoka. And those who fake knowledge and in doing so lead others astray? That's a problem exclusive to the tea ceremony, surely not something we have to guard against in the martial arts.

Maybe there are so many lessons to be learned in the dojo that we don't need to investigate other Ways or listen to the words of those who have pursued those Ways. Maybe, though, if we broaden our views on following a Way, we'll see that others who are on different paths might lead us more deeply into and farther along our own.

30

DOES IT DO WHAT IT SAYS?

"KARATE ISN'T A MARTIAL ART," I said. And that got everyone's attention. I'd been asked to come to a karate dojo and lead a seminar. The group had been working hard. We were about to stop for lunch, and as we went through some cool-down exercises, someone asked me a question about karate as a martial art—and that's when I made the comment.

Predictably, this statement, when I make it looking out on a class of karateka, will elicit some looks of confusion—and some expressions of anger. Some are wondering what on earth I'm talking about. The faces of others will darken with rage.

Here's what I went on to explain: karate is not a martial art because it was, technically speaking, not created or practiced by professional warriors. It was not the creation of a *martial* group. Neither was it meant for direct application on a battlefield. Kendo, judo, and aikido are martial arts in that they descended directly from arts that were originated by professional warriors, the samurai, arts that were meant for use in warfare. Karate can be a *combative* art. It can be an art devoted to self-defense in nonmartial situations when it is taught by those who understand and can communicate these aspects of it. Not all *fighting* arts, though, are *martial* arts. (This applies as well to kung fu and tae kwon do, to Indonesian or Thai arts, or to the fighting arts of many other countries and cultures.)

Of course, people often don't listen carefully, don't think, and sometimes don't really care to. They are quick to take offense. If I say it isn't a martial art, what they hear me saying is that it isn't effective. That's not true at all. Saying Ping-Pong isn't a contact sport is not the same thing as saying Ping-Pong isn't a sport or that it isn't challenging or worthwhile. Unfortunately, while immersing oneself in a budo is often claimed as a way of subduing the ego, for a lot of people, budo becomes the very expression of their ego. And while they may believe they are strident about defending karate, often what they are doing is defending what they believe to be an attack on their own ego.

That brings us to the subject of karate's effectiveness. Or, for that matter, the effectiveness of any budo, any fighting art. To ask if karate is "effective" is to ask half a question. The other half is crucial to a coherent answer. Effective for what? When I look at karate, or any fighting system, what I'm looking for is simple: is there consistency between what the art claims and what it demonstrably does?

If "self-defense" is purported to be a goal in your karate, there will be some factors we should look for. For example, don't tell me your dojo is primarily concerned about teaching "realistic self-defense" and then show me the class lined up in *keikogi,* training barefoot on a smooth wooden floor. If your system says it teaches you to handle conflicts or unexpected attacks, but all your paired exercises begin with an ideal distance between you and a partner, then there is a clear disparity between what you claim and what you actually do.

So-called traditionalists are often accused of looking down their noses at the currently popular mixed "martial arts" (there's that word misused again). That's generally an inaccurate accusation. Instead, those who have some knowledge of fighting arts are more likely to assign these mixed martial arts (MMA) to their proper place. They are sports, with rules. They are conducted in an artificial environment. Contestants know what to expect and have ample time to prepare for it, to dress for it, and to condition themselves for it. Does any of that apply in a survival situation involving hand-to-hand combat? No. Does that mean MMA aren't effective? Not at all. They are perfectly effective for what they are intended to do: be an exciting, challenging sport. The kata of the Japan Karate Association is beautiful to watch. Aesthetically, it is in my opinion, the most beautiful system of karate. Does it have direct, functional, practical applications for self-defense? Nope. The self-defense applications and explanations of JKA kata are simplistic, often erroneous; generally impractical. So are they ineffective? No. They are wonderfully effective for conditioning, for exercise, for the aesthetics they possess.

So, am I proposing that MMA practitioners and JKA exponents can't fight in a real situation? Not at all. I am saying that self-defense is not the primary goal of either of these activities. It is good when teachers of these systems recognize this and do not promise those who enter them that such self-defense skills are the intent of the instruction. It's bad when they do. If a JKA black belt or an MMA champion is successful in defending himself against an attack on the street, it may doubtless have something to do with his training. But that is not the *goal* of his training. At least that is not the legitimate goal of these activities. In MMA, the goals are winning bouts and building strength and suppleness. In karate, the goals may be winning in tournaments, improving one's health (physical or psychological), and developing an aesthetic awareness.

Yes, again, I know. There are MMA and JKA guys who are quite tough and who've prevailed when attacked on the street. There are golfers who've killed rattlesnakes with their clubs. No one would argue that learning to golf is a good way to learn about defending yourself from attacking reptiles. The argument remains: A combative art is judged by how well it does what it says it's supposed to do. Keeping this in mind is probably the best yardstick you can use to measure your own art and anyone else's.

31

A MASTER OF MASTERS?

THE CALLER'S QUESTION for me was simple: "Who is the best karate practitioner in the world today?" She is a writer and was working on a piece for a general interest magazine about the "best" in several sports and physical activities.

"What makes you think it isn't me?" I said. There was stillness on the line, then some stammering. I concluded she didn't get my sense of humor. Lots of people don't. So I took a different tack. "Let me ask you this," I said. "Who is the best musician in the world today?"

"Well, that's really impossible to answer," she said. "There are so many kinds of music." Exactly.

There is a natural inclination we have, to want to know the "best" of things. In some aspects of life, we can make fairly accurate assessments of these things. We know the best miler in the world: his track record is proof. In other areas, however, assigning a title like "best" is simply impossible. Additionally, when we engage in such arbitrary qualifications, we often end up clouding the issue rather than clarifying it. Most of us in the karate world understand that there are dozens and dozens of schools and systems of karate. There are so many of these for many reasons. Political or personal disagreements can lead to schisms and factionalization that result in new schools or organizations. Differences about what aspects of training should be stressed can also lead to the proliferation of karate schools. There are forms of karate that vary so dramatically in their training, in their emphasis, and in their applications that such distinctions as ascertaining the "best" among them would be obviously futile even to those who do not practice karate. How do you determine, among these very different systems and approaches, the "best"?

People outside karate often see the art as a monolithic entity. If there is kicking involved, and black belts and such, it is "karate." The same can be said of ikebana, or Japanese flower arranging. For the majority of us, if we were presented with six different arrangements, they would all look alike. Only if we were well-trained and had many years of experience could we say, "That's an arrangement in the Ikenobo style; this one is from Ohara ryu." Similarly, it takes a practiced eye to spot the differences between, say, Goju ryu and Shito ryu in karate. However slight these differences may be, though, we know they are very real. We also know what the public usually does not: that finding the best among them leads to further misunderstanding about the true nature of karate and, by extension, the true essence of budo.

"What is the highest degree of black belt awarded in karate?" is a question I remember seeing once in a trivia game. Know the answer? No you don't. There isn't one. You can start your own karate organization tomorrow and give yourself whatever "degree" of black belt you wish. You might say that, yes, you can—but your organization will lack the credibility of the established groups in Japan and elsewhere. True. So what? The measure of a karate organization's authenticity is entirely in the eye of the prospective student in this regard. Karate has been in the United States long enough and enough senior level practitioners have been produced that we do not need a connection with Japan to establish bona fides. And yes, there are those who lack such bona fides that they seek to pad their reputations with ridiculous "sixteenth"-degree black belt status. They are silly. But there is no big, central karate organization that can say such people are wrong or are violating some law. This leads us to our final point.

Recently I saw a documentary produced in the West about a karate sensei in Japan. He was described by the narrator as a "master of masters," and later on there was the note that he had been recognized as such by "the Japanese government." Okay, let's establish this: the Japanese government cares as much about the best karate teacher in Japan as the U.S. government cares about the best badminton player in America. Usually when the Japanese government's sanction is invoked in relation to karate, the reference is to what was once known as the Monbusho, or Ministry of Education, Sports, and Culture. In 2001, the Monbusho was combined with the Japanese government's department of science and technology and is now known as the Monkasho. This department oversees nearly all areas of education in Japan, choosing textbooks, setting curricula, and so on. In 1957, the Japan Karate Association applied to be recognized as an educational corporation, under Japanese law, and to be recognized as such by the Monbusho. In a very technical sense then, the JKA can be thought of as being sanctioned by the ministry, which, by extension, means the Japanese government. However, it is easy to make too much of this. Imagine if your karate group is, for example, renting space at the Riverport City Community Center. Since the center is owned by the city, you could technically say you were an "officially recognized" form of karate by Riverport. The JKA was able to satisfy the Monbusho that its curriculum and training and goals were sufficiently coherent and meaningful to be recognized by the ministry as an educational system. This is admirable to be sure. However, it says nothing about the dozens of other karate systems in Japan that simply never applied and never saw any particular advantage in such ministerial recognition.

Karate, in Japan or anywhere else in the rest of the world, like every other form of budo, is not controlled or even organized under any comprehensive umbrella committee or organization. There are several big groups that oversee—loosely—karate systems that have voluntarily joined. The World Union of Karate Organizations (WUKO) and the Federation of All-Japan Karate Organizations (FAJKO) are two of the better known of these. In a sense, these may be thought of as being the equivalent of Major League Baseball in the United States. They are corporations. Member groups participate because, in the main, membership allows for tournaments between the various systems. Think, though, of all the baseball that is played in the United States that has absolutely no connection with major league baseball. It is the same way with karate. In Japan there are literally hundreds and hundreds of small dojo that are completely independent. They don't know who the big leaders are of WUKO or FAJKO, and they don't care. If you are the president of WUKO and come to one of these dojo, they would, I'm guessing, treat you politely. But you would have no special status there. FAJKO may declare one of their members a "master." That matters little to the karate teacher who has a dozen students he teaches in a garage-sized dojo on the first floor of his home.

Doubtless it is appealing to be able to point to one person in any martial art and say, as we would for Olympic champions or marksmen or many other kinds of athletes, "He's the best." Think of it another way, though. We don't really know who is the best, so our karate or whatever budo we are pursuing becomes even more fascinating. Maybe when you began your training, your idea of the best karate teacher was the guy who could smash the biggest pile of boards. As you progressed, you began to see other attributes that you now know are more significant and worthwhile. What you think of as the best in karate says as much about you as it does the art and the person you elect to teach you. It isn't a definitive answer. But it is an intriguing one.

32

WHY NOT?

RECENTLY, AN EDITOR of mine wrote a timely and, I thought, provocative editorial for a martial arts magazine. (Never hurts to flatter an editor.) He recounted the trying circumstances of dealing with a champion of "mixed martial arts" (MMA), who was scheduled to show up at the magazine offices for a cover photo shoot. The man was apparently quite important—or at least considered himself so. He first had a flunky call to say he wouldn't be doing any action shots: he was sore from a recent bout. Then he said he'd be a "little late." It went on and on. His lackeys continued to postpone, promise, and prevaricate, causing headaches for the photographer and the magazine's staff. The shoot was eventually cancelled. The guy, needless to say, will not be appearing on the cover of that magazine any time soon. The editor used the incident in his editorial to illustrate how big egos and bad attitudes are really not conducive to success in any field. Particularly they are out of place in the martial arts.

First, let's establish that this is not a problem solely with MMA practitioners. It was around long before the first cage match or full contact bout ever began. I visited the offices of that particular magazine more than twenty years ago, right after a "traditionalist" had stormed out of the place and sat and pouted in his car for over an hour in the parking lot because the magazine staff did not address him as "Master." Another functionary to some big, self-appointed martial arts maestro once contacted the offices to lay the groundwork for a proposed visit. He sent head shots of half a dozen of the fellow's entourage to allow, he said, time for the magazine staff to memorize the faces and the accompanying titles—*renshi, shidoshi,* and so forth—of each so they could be properly addressed when they arrived. No, unfortunately, these attitudes are not uncommon in any of the activities labeled "martial arts." For me, the interesting question is this: why not?

What's wrong with behaving this way, behaving like an arrogant prima donna? Certainly we overlook it and, in fact, even celebrate this kind of behavior in many other areas. Professional athletes, entertainers, "do you know who I am?" politicians: they all routinely engage in self-centered, arrogant displays meant to establish or enforce their own sense of importance. If you haven't seen an example of boorish public behavior in a celebrity, you must not ever have turned on the news or picked up a paper. Sometimes it seems the more successful people are—or at least the more famous they are—the more abysmal their conduct. The MMA champion, the ninth-dan karate master, the inventor of a new, super-spectacularly deadly art: why should they be any different?

The roots of a prescribed "code of conduct" in the Japanese combat arts are in neo-Confucian thought. Confucius believed proper conduct was as essential to life as food or air. He believed the state was a macrocosm of the family. I am obedient to the king for the same reason I am obedient to my father. The king treats me well for the same reason my father does. Of course, this sort of philosophy was very attractive to the military leaders of feudal Japan. They imported Confucian ideas from China; demonstrating respect for one's superiors in social and political settings had an obvious advantage for Japan's rulers. It kept people in line and under control.

The second influence on the behaviors we have come to associate with budo—self-control and modesty and politeness—was, in my opinion, both a direct and an indirect consequence of the substantial number of weapons around in feudal Japan. While only those members of the samurai class could carry a long and short sword together, during most of Japan's feudal era, other classes like nonsamurai, farmers, merchants, craftsmen, carried a sword or some other edged weapon commonly. Sometimes it was for protection, other times the sword was worn to imitate the samurai, as a kind of status symbol. In any event, there were a lot of swords, and so rules of civility were established to keep the whole country from turning into a bloody mess.

The third influence was on the status of the samurai themselves. It is a ridiculous notion that these warriors always behaved graciously or courteously. We have already noted in a couple of chapters previously here that they were capable of rudeness, incredible cruelty, and callous behavior. Many of them would have been right at home with the conduct of that MMA guy. It is also true, however, that people of the nonsamurai castes looked at the warrior with some respect. Yes, the farmers raised the food, and the merchants provided the goods. But the samurai was the one who, in times of mortal danger, provided the protection that meant the difference between life and death. The warrior had skills and the will to put his life on the line. Again, certainly not in all cases, but in many instances, the samurai were aware of their position, and they acted accordingly. They behaved, sometimes anyway, as if they were worthy of the respect of others. One way in which that was done then is the same way it is done now—by showing respect in return.

It is an adage for a woman first dating a man that, if she wants his measure, she should see how he treats others who are serving him. The waiter, the taxi driver, the store clerk: the way a guy treats these people gives one insight into how he thinks of others and how he'll think of you—and ultimately how he thinks of himself. It is good advice. Maybe that is why rudeness and crass behavior have no place in the budo. Sure, it is because we have a long history of association with and influence by Confucian ethics. And a history of being involved in dangerous pursuits that lead us toward a greater awareness of our responsibilities. But we also behave ourselves and conduct ourselves with respect for others because we have a long history, too, of being respected for what we do.

33

TRY THIS AT HOME

CHILDREN'S KARATE CLASSES are frequently concluded with the stern warning that what we practice in the dojo is not for indiscriminate use. You're not supposed to "do this stuff" with friends or at home or anywhere outside the dojo, they are told. I never liked this.

To me, teaching someone to do something and then telling them not to do it is, well, a little dumb. If you are teaching someone to do something and then telling them not to do it, you'd better do some thinking about just what it is you are teaching.

"Oh, so you're saying it's okay for a kid to go home from karate class and side kick his little brother in the head? It's all right if he 'tries out' his reverse punch against a friend on the playground and breaks a nose? Throws someone and breaks an arm?"

Please reread what I just wrote. Are you teaching the children in your classes to kick people in the head or to punch others in the nose or throw them for no good reason?

"Well, no. But those kicks and punches, throws, and other such things are a part of training. That's what we're doing in a karate or a judo or an aikido class."

Yes, that's *part* of what you should be doing in those classes, of course. A big part. But it is far from the only part of a good budo

165

class, and it should not be the goal of that class. Not for kids and not for adults.

"Oh, so you want to have a discussion of philosophy instead of hard training, right? You want budo class to be like a church service or a therapy session."

Nope. There needs to be a whole lot *less* talking in dojo in my opinion. Too much time is spent talking, trying to explain things intellectually that are only adequately grasped when you learn them with your body. We often hear the adage, "Shut up and train." Good advice. But the sensei ought to be saying to himself, "Shut up and teach."

So, let's look at the fundamentals of the situation. First, we have children who, because they're children, do not always behave in mature, reasonable ways. And as children, they sense their relative powerlessness in society, and when they are given power, they sometimes abuse it—like kicking their brother in the head. Karate affords them the ability to kick like that; it is unrealistic to think they will not at least be tempted to do it. Yes, you can give them a lecture. It might work. What I think is more effective, and what I learned when I was a child practicing karate, is for teachers and seniors in the dojo to be role models. The leadership in the dojo do not go around indiscriminately kicking others in the head. They don't even play at it. When we are kicking, it is under the special circumstances of training. We reinforce the idea we are doing something special in the uniforms we wear only in the dojo. The attitude in the dojo reinforces it. It is not "playtime" in the dojo, ever. The atmosphere is friendly and relaxed, but it is serious. Karate and other budo do not get treated the way we might treat, say, an afternoon fun program at the Y. The budo are different. We do well to recognize this and approach our own training and the teaching of others, especially children, with that in mind. Were I a grade-school basketball coach, I wouldn't mind if one of my players shot hoops with his brother at home. Were I teaching karate, I would mind very much if that child treated the art like he would a basketball game. That difference has to be made clearly and consistently. Think of it this way: don't use a budo class as entertainment for a kiddie birthday party, and you won't have to worry so much about it being misused in other ways.

Second, if all we are teaching is kicking and punching and throwing, we cannot be surprised if that is the lesson children get from class. If children in a martial arts class get positive attention from being aggressive or for winning tournaments or being the center of attention, they will learn from that. They will learn what is valued in the dojo and seek to identify with those values. If, on the other hand, self-control and poise and humility are highlighted, those are the values the child is going to esteem and emulate. If the teacher struts about, uniform festooned with insignia, demanding to be called "master," children in the class are going to assume power is primarily for boosting one's ego and status. If the child sees a teacher who is unassuming and who trains alongside the class, who readily admits his own weaknesses and shows others he's working on them, the kid learns to behave accordingly. If the curriculum changes to meet whatever popular interest has been sparked by a martial arts movie or an Olympic competition, the child learns his art doesn't have any fixed concepts or ideals and is, instead, a product. If the art is taught with consistency and within the framework of what has been taught in the past, the kid in that budo class learns to see himself as a part in something larger and more important than himself. There are a lot of lessons taught in the dojo that have little directly to do with hitting and throwing people. Integrity, respect for other people, dignity, and honesty: they aren't in the kata or in freestyle exercises. But they're in the dojo, too—or they are not. And there are consequences, either way, for those training there.

Sure, it is absurdly idealistic to think that no matter what we do to influence or direct them, that children will always behave appropriately. We have to keep an eye on them and look for behavior that might demonstrate aggressiveness or a need to show off or strike out in frustration. And if we see that, we do need to talk to them and to their parents. However, if the budo are the Ways many of us think they are, then the best approach for getting others—especially children—to walk the Ways is to lead by example.

34

WHAT'S WRONG WITH
THE JAPANESE?

AN ATTENDEE, having to leave a large aikido seminar early, had ducked out during a break and, on his way to the parking lot, saw the guest instructor, who was by himself at the rear of the gymnasium, smoking. The student approached and excused himself, noting he was leaving early and thanking the instructor for coming. The Japanese instructor, one of the highest-ranking aikido teachers in the United States, head of a national organization, and personal student of the art's founder, glanced at the student, blew smoke in his direction, and without a single word consciously turned his back on the stunned young man.

A jujutsu teacher at a large public demonstration was display-ing self-defense moves against multiple opponents. He whirled to face an attacker at his rear, one of his own students, and unleashed a spearhand thrust to the student's throat. The Japanese teacher's balance and control were both poor. He drove his fingertips right into the student's throat. The student collapsed, unable to breathe and struggling to remain conscious. He was in real danger of dying. As other students rushed to his assistance, the teacher glared, hands on his hips, and complained loudly—and falsely—"He moved right into it!"

A Japanese karate instructor is a frequent sight on the downtown streets in the U.S. city where he teaches, strolling about wearing a replica cap of an Imperial Japanese Army officer.

A senior student of another internationally renowned Japanese karate teacher in the West had worked for years to create a distinctive method of teaching that incorporated kata with self-defense drills. Proudly, he demonstrated it to his teacher—who presented it a few months later at a seminar, claiming it as his own.

I can keep going. For a long time. If the reader has much experience in the martial arts, he can add his own such stories. Indeed, the question is not how many tales of outrage we can tell. It is this: why are so many Japanese martial arts instructors such contemptible, horribly ill-behaving jerks?

Now, hold on. Let's establish a couple of matters right away: There are plenty of jerks in positions of teaching authority in the budo who come from every race and ethnicity known to man. Martial arts seem to draw a lot of people who have emotional or psychological problems, and far too many of them hang around long enough to attain positions as teachers. The various psychoses and neuroses of these instructors from both East and West are on wide and varied display. This is not our subject. More specifically, we are looking at the phenomenon of those Japanese teachers who have come to the West and who demonstrate disgusting, thoughtless, even immoral behavior and who seem to treat their students more like annoying distractions than as the source of income those students are. And let's establish that, in getting uncomfortably close to half a century of budo training, I have had many, many juniors, seniors, and teachers who are Japanese. I am constantly active in the expatriate Japanese community where I live and spend considerable time there, both professionally and avocationally. Japanese, both in and out of the martial arts, have profoundly influenced me, and in many ways I can never repay them. I make much of my living writing about aspects of Japanese culture. I have nothing personal against Japanese or Japanese society.

Okay, so I'm acknowledging that uncivil, even vile, behavior is not the exclusive domain of Japanese budo teachers. So why accentuate their failings? Why does it seem I am holding them to a different standard than Western martial arts teachers? I am not. I condemn all bad behavior in and out of the dojo by martial arts teachers, and it is deplorable whenever it occurs. I have written thousands of words about it in this book alone. I am focusing on this behavior among Japanese instructors here, however, for two reasons. First, many Westerners have expectations of Japanese instructors they may not have for non-Japanese teachers. The budo, after all, came from Japan. It is natural to believe the Japanese would have a deeper understanding of budo's goals and exhibit a high standard of behavior. (I did not say that such a belief is valid. Or reasonable. Only that it is natural, and common.) And the Japanese teachers themselves, in many cases, have buttressed that perception, inaccurate though demonstrably it is. Indeed, Japanese teachers of high rank, teachers at the heads of virtually every major budo organization, have presented themselves as "masters," as unquestionable authority figures. Non-Japanese members of these organizations have been told to their faces that they cannot really, truly, understand the profundities of Japanese budo. They have been told this after devoting decades to those budo. That these people continue to train under such nonsense is incredible to me. But it happens. Indeed, the majority of Japanese-born teachers who act as the heads of budo organizations in the West have been shown the way to the pedestal by credulous, unquestioning Western students. In most instances, however, the Japanese teachers were not at all hesitant in hopping up onto that pedestal.

So how did it happen? As neither a historian nor a psychologist, let me nevertheless offer a brief history and psychological perspective: Japanese budo, or martial arts, were, until the modern era, the province of a professional warrior class: the samurai. The businessman or farmer, the average Japanese, had little interest in combative arts other than sumo, which was widely practiced by all classes in feudal Japan. What we think of as "martial arts" in Japan—karate-do, judo, kendo, and aikido—were not some ancient part of traditional Japanese life. In truth, they evolved rapidly after the end of the feudal period, when Japan adopted a constitutional monarchy and modernized as a nation. As Japan emerged into the modern era, its increased wealth made a higher standard of living for the average Japanese. Many of these average Japanese were able for the first time to pursue hobbies or avocations. The budo became popular with people from all walks of life. As time went on, at least two changes pertinent to our topic occurred. One, the harsh realities of feudal life, including the rule of the samurai, became a little fuzzy in retrospect and attained a glow of the nostalgic. Two, Japan's rise as a military and economic power began to have a powerful influence on the Japanese. Japan has always viewed itself as a special place—there is even a term, *nihonjin-ron,* to self-describe this sense of uniqueness. Given the rapid and successful modernization of the country, however, this attitude took a dark and explosive turn. From Shinto to sushi, everything in the sphere of Japanese culture and civilization was employed by Japan's politicians and military to advance the notion of Japan's greatness and moral rectitude. Japan was, its citizens were constantly told during the 1920s and 1930s, destined to rule the world, to unite the "eight corners" of the earth under a single—Japanese—"roof."

By the early 1930s, Japan had become one of the more militaristic societies on earth. Remember though, that this militarism was not the traditional feudal martial ethos of the samurai. It was informed more by Prussian and other Western concepts of the military that had been imported by Japanese leaders eager to copy the military success of Germany. The Japanese soldiers who invaded Korea in 1895—and who went to Manchuria in 1931—believed they were the modern incarnation of the now-noble samurai. They were not. Their fanaticism and rigid "gung-ho" enthusiasms were a theatrical imitation of the lifestyle of the average samurai, who, as hereditary warriors, would have held such mentalities in some contempt. (The militarists were closer in spirit to those same samurai-wannabes we talked about earlier, in some of today's budo dojo.) This, it is no co-incidence, is the world into which most of the Japanese budo leaders living and teaching in the United States matured. There is simply no doubt it affected them deeply. We can read tales of karate training at universities during this time, of incredible brutality and "do or die" attitudes. Obedience to authority was a sign of patriotism. Unquestioned loyalty was proof of sincerity. Even the most devoted karate student today, for example, would be shocked at the levels of commitment and dedication, fueled by nationalist zealotry, of the average Japanese university karateka of that day.

Of course, we know how it all ended. Japan, for the first time in its existence as a civilization, had conquerors walking about freely on its soil. For decades, the Japanese had been indoctrinated in the superiority, the invincibility, of all things Japanese. They were faced, in 1945, with a very different, very harsh reality. The majority of Japanese who came to the West to teach budo in the late 1950s and early 1960s endured significant emotional and psychological damage at a crucial time in their youth, in the 1940s. Young men of any culture take pride in strength and power. To have that stripped away as dramatically as the end of World War II did in Japan would not have been easy. The first Japanese martial arts instructors came to America, I think it is safe to say, with some decidedly conflicting emotions.

Many Americans took it for granted that the first real wave of Japanese teachers who appeared in the West in the 1960s were "masters." They looked the part. They had talents no one could match in the West. In truth, most Japanese instructors who came to the West were young and, while well trained, they had relatively little experience, on average, in teaching. Certainly they didn't have much experience teaching outside the still-insular culture of Japan. They had a rough go of it. Homesick, unaccustomed to Western food, often so poor they were sleeping on the dojo floor, they struggled with a foreign culture and language. They were trying to impart skills and knowledge almost completely unknown in the West. It was not easy.

Things were complicated considerably by the Western romanticization of karate, judo, and the budo in general. Westerners also had vastly exaggerated ideas about the skill of these new teachers and no idea of how to treat those teachers. From a Western perspective, the arrival of Japanese professional budo teachers was greeted much the same way Indian yogis and swamis from India were treated when they arrived en masse in in the United States in the 1960s. The West has long had a fascination with the East and with Japan in particular. These young, talented Japanese came bringing what looked like near-miraculous powers. Credulous Western students idolized them. They could not or would not see any flaws in these teachers. They made excuses for bad behavior from Japanese teachers, or ignored it. Where in Japan a senior instructor or some other authority figure would have stepped in when the students did not protest, in the United States and elsewhere, the Japanese instructors were without any sort of oversight. They answered, in terms of their deportment day to day, to no one. (An exception was in Hawaii, where many of the students were fluent in both the language and the native culture of Japan. There were several instances in the 1960s when these students went over the heads of misbehaving sensei and complained directly to organization leaders in Japan—and got satisfactory results.)

The average Western student also had almost no perspective on budo during this period of the arts' mainstream introduction. When Japanese teachers asked what seemed to be extraordinary efforts—standing barefoot practicing kicks in the snow, smashing bricks with one's forehead, paying for being beaten ("to forge your spirit!")—the beginner karateka in Ohio had no way of knowing if this wasn't normal in karate dojo in Osaka. Now we laugh at "bow to your sensei!" For many in the previous generation of Western martial artists, however, that would have been the way of things in a typical class.

It is worth reiteration: I am not a psychologist. It doesn't take a PhD, though, to see the potential for abuse in the situation we've just outlined. Look at it this way: For many relatively young Japanese men, their country's military defeat was also a matter of personal emotional devastation. They were suddenly in charge of large groups of people who had been, only a short time ago, reviled as barbarian enemies. (A Japanese friend who grew up during this period told me that officers had come to his grade school during the war to explain that if the United States invaded Japan, the Americans had a plan to forcibly breed Japanese women with black GIs, the better to produce a race of intelligent and strong slaves.) I do not wish to imply that every newly arrived Japanese aikido or karate-do teacher sat at the front of his class in Omaha or Pittsburgh and thought, "At last! A chance to humiliate the conquerors!" But the scars of the Second World War were still very fresh. Abuses did occur, as they continue to. I recall vividly hearing an aikido teacher during the 1960s, who was speaking Japanese to another instructor, say, after he injured a student while throwing him: "When are these stupid foreigners going to realize they can't do real budo?"

The first generation of Japanese martial arts teachers in the West was also frustrated at the inability to communicate. It was a limitation imposed not only from lack of conversance in the language but also in the inability to adequately describe some of the elements of budo. These teachers were frustrated as well to have questions presented by their Western students, questions for which they had no good answers. As most readers will know, the prevalent Japanese method of teaching is to demonstrate and to have the student copy without question or without thinking much about the process at all. So in dojo in Cleveland or Sarasota, there were—and continue to be—exchanges like this: "Sensei, when we make an elbow strike, should our hand be open or closed?" "Closed." "Why?" "Because I said so!" In reality, the "master" was probably trying to remember how his teacher had done it. Or, if he did know, he was faced with the sudden realization that he had never asked his own teacher why the strike was done the way it was. In any case, not being sure of the answer can be embarrassing, and worse, it can be interpreted as creating a question of the teacher's authority and competence. The status of any teacher in Japan has always tended to be higher than we afford teachers in the

United States. A question, even a sincere one, could easily be interpreted as a challenge, as an affront. The very fact that you are asking a question is a commentary on the teacher's inability to teach. "How can you not understand—I just showed you!" Here, the frustration is compounded by the realization of the teacher that he in fact does not have all the answers. It occurs to him, perhaps, when he is not able to answer every question instantly and authoritatively, that maybe he doesn't really belong on that pedestal after all.

All of these factors have worked to create the situation we have today. It is important to realize that the situation is not as awful as we are painting it here: we are focusing on the bad, highlighting it, to make a point. There are Japanese sensei all over the West who have gone to the trouble of assimilating, learning the language of their adopted homes, working constantly to improve communication with their students, being good leaders and teachers. Still, it is naive not to recognize that a problem exists. And so, what can you do about it? Consider these suggestions, ones that apply equally to a dojo or budo organization whether it is run by a Japanese or by a Westerner:

Japanese budo, all of them, depend substantially on Japanese culture. I cannot state this strongly enough. That said, just because an individual is racially Japanese does not mean he understands Japanese culture—particularly the culture of Japanese budo—or that he can transmit it. I have met several Western martial artists who have spent decades in Japan and who understand the ethos of Japanese budo better than most modern Japanese sensei.

Do not assume that just because the teacher in the dojo or the head of the organization is Japanese that there is, implicitly or explicitly, some kind of "authenticity" there. It is true that most serious budo dojo and organizations have close links with Japan. Yet often now a non-Japanese teacher will have established those links. Plenty of Western martial arts teachers have matured and reached positions of authority, and they do not need a Japanese instructor to "validate" their experience or expertise.

Watch to see how the teacher conducts himself, how he relates to the students. I have never met or even heard of a teacher in Japan who does not socialize with his students outside the dojo, going out for a beer after training or attending holiday parties or taking at least some interest in interacting with the families of his students. If the teacher does not ever seem to be able to relax, if he has one persona—The Guy In Charge—that never changes, it's not a good sign that he is a well-balanced individual.

If you can, find out what sort of groups or friendships the teacher has outside the dojo. This is critical. A teacher whose only relationships are through his teaching is like a person who only has a parental relationship with a child and who does not regularly interact with other people. Imagine if everyone with whom you socialized was under your control, if you related to everyone in your life as you would with your own young child. Not very healthy, right? The teacher who, in addition to being "sensei" in the dojo, is also active in the community or in other social areas tends to have a more balanced self-image. I once stayed with a karate teacher whose neighbors addressed him not as "Master" or "Sensei" but as "Kaz" and who ribbed him about his always-broken lawn mower. Those are the sort of relationships that keep things in perspective for a high-ranked instructor.

Look for a dojo in which the majority of members are not only adults but are also educated and mature and who do not appear to be in need of a "guru" or father figure, someone with all the answers who habitually treats them as children or fawning acolytes. There are some people, unfortunately too, who would rather train with a poorly skilled Japanese teacher than a highly qualified Westerner. In these instances, they are looking more for an image and less for the substance that is budo.

Use independent information when you are confronted with things that appear wrong. There is a dismayingly large amount of silliness and misinformation in books and on the Internet, to be sure. Yet there is also a lot of very good advice and knowledge. If something's going on in your dojo that you have questions about, there are forums where you can post those questions and usually get a variety of answers that can give you a better perspective.

As we mentioned in an earlier chapter and in a slightly different but related context, don't abandon your common sense. Yes, Japan and Japanese culture are different from the West and its cultures. Even so, a teacher who is making romantic advances on the wife of a student is an immoral jerk, whether he's Japanese or Western. Even in those instances where differences do exist, they should not be used as an excuse for otherwise unjustifiable behavior. In the discussion earlier, on budo etiquette, I gave an example of a judoka winning a bout by taking advantage of an outstretched hand offered to "help" an opponent get back to his feet after an inconclusive throw. That is a legitimate strategy if we remember that we're talking about a martial art and that we must have some sense of awareness. It does not mean I am justified if I knock you down in a judo or karate bout, and then stomp on your jaw when you are on the ground. Deliberately inflicted injuries, emotional cruelty, insincerity: these are the signs of the sociopath, in the East as well as in the West.

There is probably no healthier sign of a good teacher than one who can laugh at himself and who, while he has established himself as the leader and the model, will cheerfully admit his own mistakes and limitations. I have on frequent occasions been in the company of budo teachers, highly ranked ones, and had the opportunity to speak frankly and directly with them. When I do, I always, sooner or later, ask the same question: "What are you working on in your training?" It'd be fun to have a video compilation of their responses. Some look at me as if I had just asked them to saw off one of their own limbs. A few have been insulted. "I am a sensei. Who do you think you are to ask me that?" "Yes," I reply. "You are a sensei. But you're not *my* sensei. I've met and trained with other sensei at your level. I respect you just like I do them. But aside from that, you're no different. *That's* who I am to ask you that." Some, however, will happily tell me where they think they are weak and on what particular skills they are trying to develop. These are the sorts of teachers I would be willing to call "Sensei"—whether they are Japanese or Western.

Glossary

aikido. Literally the "Way of Uniting Ki," aikido is a modern Japanese martial art focusing on the use of throws, pinning techniques, and locks, and integrating specific movements to control an opponent.

aikidoka. A person who practices aikido.

aratameshi. Testing a sword or other blade by repeatedly striking it against a hard object until it either bends or breaks.

bo. A wooden staff.

budo. The Japanese martial Ways.

budoka. A generic term for those who practice any of the Japanese martial Ways.

bushi. Another term for samurai.

bushido. The "Way of the Warrior." A generalized term used to describe the conduct and philosophy of the professional warrior class in Japan during the feudal period there.

chado. The Japanese tea ceremony.

chadoka. A person who practices chado.

daimyo. A lord or lords under the feudal system of premodern Japan.

damashi. "Spirit." Damashi is the attitude or will expressed by someone and it is an indication of their commitment.

dan-i. The ranking system used in most modern Japanese martial arts. The familiar "black belt" and the system of awarding colored belts are part of the dani-i method of grading participants in an art. Dan-i methods of grading include kyu and dan ranks that indicate the level of skill of the practitioner.

den-i. A method of ranking or licensing typically used by classical martial arts, which employs scrolls or written licenses to recognize rank and teaching authority.

debana-waza. Techniques that are initiated rather than responsive.

do. A Way. *Do* is a suffix applied to indicate that an art professes to have philosophical goals as well as technical aims.

go. One of the world's oldest board games, invented in China and developed in Japan and elsewhere, go involves the taking and keeping of areas of the game board and capturing or neutralizing the territory of the opponent.

goju ryu. A popular system of karate with both Japanese and original Okinawan versions.

hakama. A pleated skirt, once worn by Japanese, now most commonly seen worn in some forms of budo.

hamon. Expulsion from a ryu.

hanbo. A "half-bo," the hanbo is a staff of usually around three feet or less in length.

hansoku-gachi. To win because of the violation of a rule by one's opponent.

ha-suji. The cutting angle of a sword or blade.

hono embu. Demonstrations that are meant, symbolically at least, to be performed before the spirits of one's ancestors in an art.

iaido. A martial Way devoted to unsheathing the sword, cutting (against an imaginary opponent), then returning the blade to the scabbard.

ikebana. The Japanese art of flower arranging.

ikenobo. A traditional style of flower arranging.

Japan Karate Association. A particular system of karate, popular in Japan and throughout the world.

jo. A staff that is longer than three feet but shorter than six feet in length.

judoka. A practitioner of judo.

jutte. A forked truncheon, carried principally by law enforcement officers in premodern Japan, used for disarming sword-wielding opponents and as a symbol of status for the officer.

kachi-nuki. To advance in a contest by winning successive victories.

kachi-toru. See *kachi-nuki.*

kado. Another term for the Japanese art of flower arranging. *Kado* means literally, the "Way of flowers."

karateka. A practitioner of karate.

kata. Dynamic exercises, either solo or with a partner, in which one trains in the fundamentals of an art. Kata are essentially the grammar of an art, a way of teaching and reinforcing its principles.

katana. The Japanese sword.

keikogi. The uniform worn for martial arts practice.

kihon. The basics or fundamentals of an art.

kirigami. A certificate indicating either rank or one's official license to teach an art.

kiri-sute gomen. The legal right of the samurai to kill those of other castes. More popular in fiction than in historical reality. See also *tsuji-kiri.*

kobo ichi. The strategy that defense and attack must be simultaneous.

kumite. Free exchanges of technique. The term is usually confined to karate.

kusarigama. A sickle and weighted chain, used as a weapon. The kusarigama was not an adaptation of the farmer's implement but rather was specifically designed as a weapon.

kutsu-bako. A box or shelf where shoes are placed before entering a dojo.

kyu-dan. Ranking systems that typically use belts or other visible methods to indicate rank. Most modern budo systems employ kyu-dan. See also *dan-i.*

kyudo. The traditional art of Japanese archery.

kyusho. Vital targets on the human body.

makimono. Wrapped scrolls. Makimono can be artwork or calligraphy. In martial arts, makimono usually is some kind of license awarded to a practitioner.

menkyo. A license that allows one to teach or represent an art. A menkyo may come in the form of a scroll or makimono, or a paper.

menkyo-kaiden. A term of rank or authority used in some martial art lineages to indicate that a person has a full understanding of the techniques, strategies, and philosophy of the art.

mokuroku. Literally a "catalogue," *mokuroku* refers to those areas of an art that a person is allowed to teach. A mokuroku can also simply be a listing of the techniques of an art.

naginata-do. The Japanese art of the glaive or halberd.

nihonjin-ron. A word sometimes used by Japanese and others to describe the uniqueness of Japan, its people, and culture.

nunchaku. A twin-hinged instrument that is used as a weapon in many Okinawan fighting systems.

Ohara ryu. A school of Japanese flower arranging.

oji-waza. Techniques employed in an art.

osu. A rough, very informal greeting, usually confined to young Japanese men, which has become, for obscure reasons, a catchall response in martial arts.

randori. Free practice in which participants exchange techniques without any prior agreement as to what they will be. The word is usually confined to judo and aikido.

renshi. A title or rank, usually indicating some level of teaching authority in a martial art.

rokushaku-bo. A staff, approximately six feet in length, used in various martial arts.

ronin. A person of the samurai class who has, for one reason or another, lost the sponsorship of his lord.

ryu. A system or lineage of an art.

saho. Etiquette.

seiryoku zenyo. A favorite aphorism of the founder of Kodokan judo, Jigoro Kano, which means "maximum efficiency with minimum effort."

seiza. A method of sitting, resting the buttocks on the heels.

sen no sen. To take the initiative in an attack.

Sengoku jidai. The period of Japanese history, circa 1400–1600, marked by internecine warfare throughout the country.

shaku. A length, taken from a traditional Japanese means of measuring, that equals 30.3 centimeters or 11.93 inches. It is sometimes roughly measured as the length between the wrist and elbow.

shiai. A contest.

shiaijo. The area where a contest is held.

shibireru. The sensation—or more accurately, the lack thereof—when one's feet and lower limbs become numb after sitting in seiza for a long time.

shibu. A group of people practicing an art.

shibu-cho. The leader of a shibu.

shidoshi. A rank or title used by some martial arts, generally indicating some level of teaching authority.

Shinkage ryu. A classical school of swordsmanship and martial strategy.

Shito ryu. A system of karate with both Japanese and Okinawan influences.

shodan. The first of the dan grades in the dan-i system of ranking; it is usually symbolized by the awarding of a black belt.

shodo. The art of Japanese calligraphy.

Shotokan Karate International. An organization founded in 1977 by Hirokazu Kanazawa to further his interpretation of the Shotokan system of karate.

shucho embu. A public demonstration of a martial art.

suemono-giri. Cutting a fixed object with the sword. See also *tameshigiri.*

suigetsu. "Water and moon." The phrase describes a mental equanimity where one's consciousness is so placid and calm it can perfectly perceive and reflect events much the same way as a still pool of water reflects the image of the moon overhead.

sumotori. A practitioner of sumo.

sun. A unit of length, equal to 30.30 millimeters or 1.193 inches, according to a traditional method of Japanese measurement. It is defined, roughly, by the distance between the fingertip and its first joint.

sun-dome. To "stop" at the distance of a single sun. See *sun.* The ability to control one's attack, stopping just short of making contact.

takabakari. An old, traditional method of measurement in premodern Japan.

tameshigiri. Cutting a fixed target or object with a sword to test the capability of the weapon or the swordsman. Technically, *tameshigiri* is used primarily to describe the cutting of a human corpse, once a common way of testing. Today, the word is used interchangeably with *suemono-giri.*

tameshiwari. Breaking objects with fists, feet, or other parts of the body, to demonstrate skill and power. Tameshiwari is the familiar "board breaking" often seen in karate demonstrations.

tanbo. A shortened version of the staff.

tatami. Woven straw mats measuring approximately three by six feet, which are traditional floor coverings in Japan and are also used to express standard measurements of a house or room size.

Tatsumi ryu. A classical school of martial arts dating back to the early sixteenth century.

te. Literally "hand," the word refers to several empty-handed Okinawan percussive arts.

Toda ryu. A classical school of Japanese martial arts, comprehensive in curriculum, that employs a number of different weapons in its training and practice.

tsuji-kiri. A term to describe killings, usually by samurai, carried out often against unarmed members of other classes in feudal Japan. These killings might be precipitated by insults, real or imagined, against the swordsman, or simply to test the quality of a weapon or a technique. *Tsuji-kiri* means literally "cutting at a crossroads."

Urasenke. The largest and oldest of the formal schools of the tea ceremony.

waza ari. A half-point, used in scoring competitive judo matches.

zanshin. "Lingering mind." Zanshin describes the state of continued awareness of the surroundings, one's opponent, and so forth, after the conclusion of a technique or encounter.

Printed in the United States
by Baker & Taylor Publisher Services